Microbiology for the Public Health

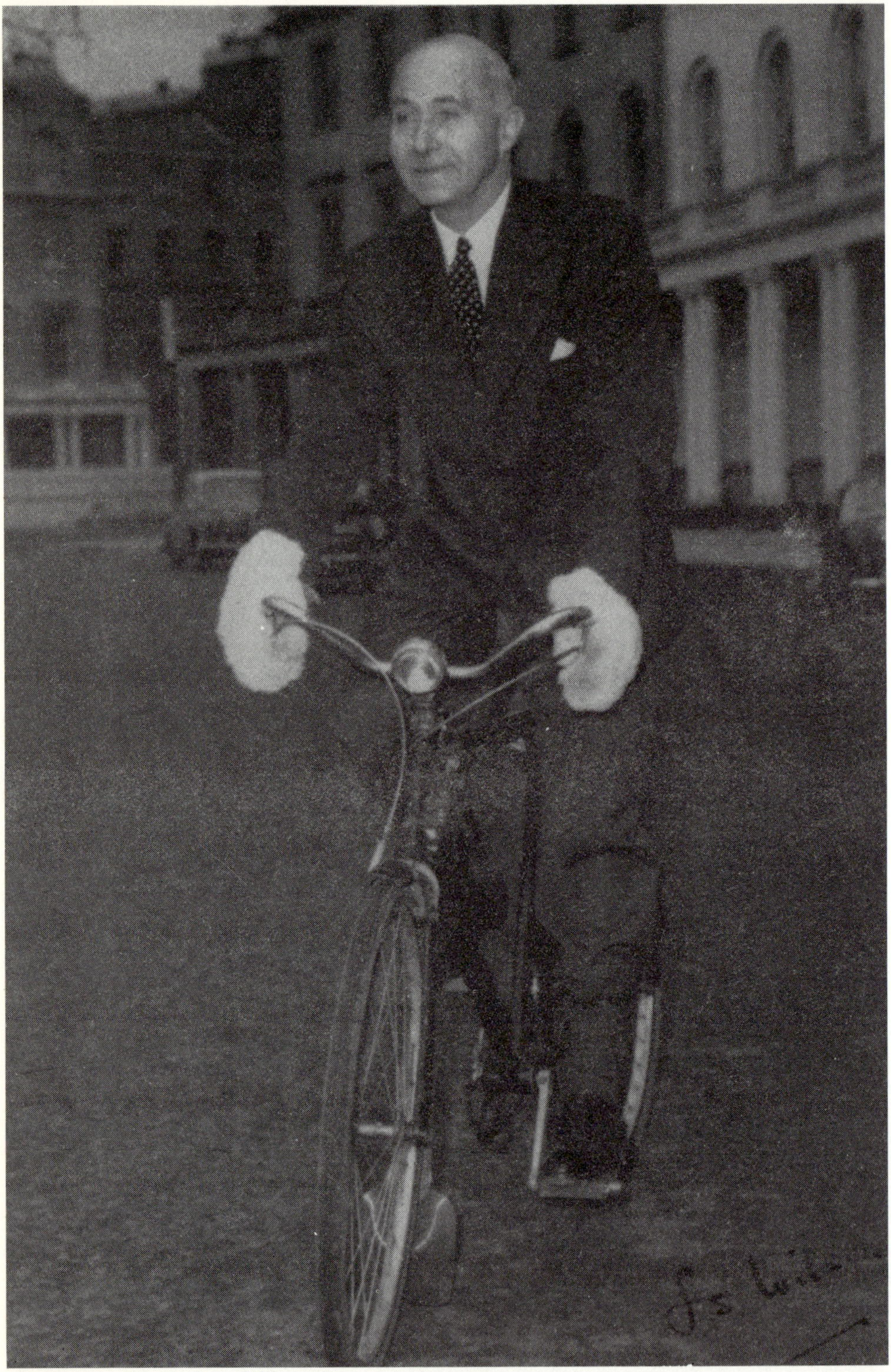

Frontispiece Sir Graham Wilson.

Microbiology for the Public Health

The Evolution of the Public Health Laboratory Service 1939–1980

by

R. E. O. Williams

London **1985**

Public Health Laboratory Service

Published by the Public Health Laboratory Service,
61 Colindale Avenue, London NW9 5DF

ISBN (hardback) 0 901 14415 0
ISBN (paperback) 0 901 14418 5

Typeset by Inforum Ltd, Portsmouth
and printed in Great Britain by
Devon and Sidmouth Printing Group, Exeter, England

To
G. S. W.
for his 90th birthday:
10 September 1985

Preface

The last 50 years have seen great changes in the prevalence and behaviour of microbial diseases and enormous growth in our ability to recognize them, to identify the causal agents, to trace their spread, and to initiate control. In Britain, the Public Health Laboratory Service (PHLS) and its predecessor, the Emergency Public Health Laboratory Service (EPHLS), have had a central role in these developments. In this essay I have attempted to recount the way in which the Service has evolved in response to the changing epidemiological scene, and the way in which it has been instrumental in bringing about some of these changes. This evolution has transformed what was originally a traditional public health microbiological service, directed to the control of infectious diseases in the community, into one that regards "public health" as embracing also the microbiology of the great variety of infective diseases seen in hospital. At the same time, the changes in the responsibilities of the community physicians have meant that many of the functions of the old-style medical officer of health have had to be assumed by the laboratory service. These developments are of intrinsic historical interest, but many of the fundamental changes have occurred in other countries, which have responded in different ways. It is hoped that an account of the development of the services in England and Wales may be of use in studies of parallel developments elsewhere.

I have ended my account around 1980, principally because 1979 had seen a substantial change in some characteristics of the PHLS as a consequence of the addition of the Ministry of Defence's Microbiological Research Establishment to the PHLS Board's responsibilities. In any case, the 1970s saw the culmination of the development that started in the early 1950s for truly close integration of the activities of the PHLS with those of the hospital microbiology services.

Plush, February 1985 R.E.O.W.

Acknowledgements and Apologies

After Sir Graham Wilson retired from the post of Director of the Public Health Laboratory Service in 1963, he wrote "Some historical notes on the formation and development of the Public Health Laboratory Service, 1938–1963", and this document provides an invaluable key to the relevant official papers as well as including a great deal of information not recorded elsewhere. I am very greatly indebted to it. I have consulted the original papers referred to by Sir Graham, and also the relevant Medical Research Council files for the period when the Council was concerned with the administration of the Service. Other sources that have been used include various published accounts of the Service, the minutes and papers of the PHLS Board and the Staff Committee, and the Annual Reports of the Medical Research Council, the PHLS, and the Chief Medical Officer of the Ministry of Health, later the Department of Health and Social Security. I have also used an analysis by Sir Graham and Miss Madeleine Barry of a survey that was being conducted just before the outbreak of war by Dr Candler, of the Ministry of Health, on the laboratory facilities available in England and Wales for the control of communicable diseases in the community. These records have been supplemented by personal recollections of my own, and of past and present members of the staff of the Service and others. The writing of near-contemporary history is hazardous and, as well as offering thanks to all those who have helped me with information, comments and corrections, I must offer apologies to all those whose contributions I have had to omit, or have simply overlooked.

Contents

Origins in the 1930s

In the introduction to his report "On the state of the public health" for 1937, the Chief Medical Officer of the Ministry of Health contrasted the then current situation with that a century earlier, when ". . . infectious disease . . . rioted uncontrolled to a large extent through England"; yet, seen from a viewpoint in the 1980s, the "classical" epidemic diseases were, in 1937, still widely spread and much in evidence. It was a year when a waterborne typhoid fever epidemic at Croydon affected over 300 persons and there were in total 2151 notifications of enteric fever with 206 deaths. There were over 61,000 cases of diphtheria (with 2963 deaths), 1750 deaths from whooping cough and 349 from scarlet fever; deaths from tuberculosis totalled 28,529 and it was estimated that some 40 per cent of the cows in dairy herds were infected with tuberculosis. Only perhaps for gonorrhoea (34,347 new cases reported from clinics) and food poisoning (with only 94 outbreaks reported) do the figures now seem modest. The Chief Medical Officer stressed the need for urgent notification to the local medical officer of health of food-poisoning outbreaks, including those in hospitals (a plea still familiar in the 1980s), to enable concurrent bacteriological investigations to be made.

Laboratory services for public health

The Ministry of Health had a small Bacteriological Laboratory, inherited from the Local Government Board in 1919, situated in Endell Street in central London. In this laboratory Dr W.M. Scott had for some years been applying the serotyping scheme developed by Bruce White and Kauffmann to the study of salmonella food poisoning. This was almost entirely a reference service and the laboratory staff did not participate in field investigations of food poisoning. They had, however, established a reputation both for the excellence of their work and the readiness with which they would help others. In the same laboratory, F. Griffith had developed a serotyping system for haemolytic streptococci and, with the laboratory's third medical officer, V.D. Allison, had collaborated in some seminal investigations of cross-infection in scarlet fever wards.

In London public health laboratory services were provided by seven group laboratories run by the London County Council and also the Camberwell laboratory, which had been started in 1891 with the appointment of Dr E.C. Bousfield as Municipal Bacteriologist. (Bousfield's son was later to direct this laboratory, which was absorbed into the PHLS in 1958.) In addition, there were two or three substantial private laboratories, including the long-established Clinical Research Association, while a number of the teaching hospitals, and the Lister Institute of Preventive Medicine, offered a limited service in the area of public health bacteriology.

Outside London, Dr Candler's survey of public health facilities in England and Wales in 1939, which is known to be incomplete, recorded the existence of 32 county or municipal laboratories. (The county and municipal authorities had largely separate health responsibilities.) There were also seven university departments which incorporated public health bacteriological laboratories, in many cases long established and with a high reputation. In Manchester, for example, Sheridan Delépine, appointed to the chair of pathology in 1891, soon commenced public health bacteriology and continued to provide a service for many years; furthermore, he was able to earn sufficient fees to give great support to the university department and indeed to pay a substantial contribution towards the cost of the new laboratory opened in York Place in 1905.

Delépine's successor, in 1921, was W.W.C. Topley, who was later to play such an important part in conceiving and setting up the EPHLS. Delépine's ideas were also carried to Bristol where one of his juniors, I. Walker Hall, was appointed Professor of Pathology and set up a public health bacteriology department which continued until 1958 as a part of the university department, latterly under R.H. Parry, who was both Medical Officer of Health for Bristol and Professor of Preventive Medicine, as well as being in charge of the laboratory. In Liverpool, too, the city had appointed a Corporation Bacteriologist, R.W. (later Sir Rubert) Boyce, who held the chair of pathology in the university; the "City Laboratory and University School of Hygiene" continued with public health bacteriology until 1955.

Several of the county council or municipal laboratories also had a long history. In Cardiff a public health laboratory was established as a joint venture by the city and the Glamorgan County Council in 1898. The Camberwell initiative in appointing a municipal bacteriologist in 1891 has already been mentioned. Kent had a laboratory from about 1911; Bradford from about 1919. Health authorities that did not have their own laboratories made various arrangements for the examination of public health specimens, often with local hospital pathologists, for some of whom this work generated a significant part of their income.

By 1937 many hospitals either had pathology laboratories in which bacteriological tests were carried out, or had made arrangements to have them done elsewhere. Patients with infectious diseases were generally nursed in special isolation or fever hospitals and were, except in the larger cities, under the clinical care of the medical officer of health or one of his staff. The diagnostic laboratory work for the patients in isolation hospitals was done in the laboratories offering public health bacteriological services.

Despite the substantial number of laboratories that were working in 1937, and the high standard of work in many of them, the arrangements had serious limitations and drawbacks. The service in different parts of the country was very uneven and the laboratories were all independent; the only formal opportunities for collating results from different areas were those offered by the very small Ministry laboratory and by the few epidemiologically oriented medical officers in the Ministry itself. The university and the hospital departments, and the private laboratories, all had to charge fees to the practitioners or health authorities requesting work, and in many cases this must have acted to restrain the amount of laboratory work to a level below that needed for the proper investigation of outbreaks of infection, or indeed often for the proper management of individual patients. To a very large extent the laboratories provided a "postal" service, receiving specimens through the mail, and though the postal services were often quicker in 1937 than in 1980 it was manifestly unsatisfactory for specimens from Southampton, for example, to be examined in Birmingham, or those from Exeter, Yorkshire, and even parts of Scotland, to be tested in London (Wilson, 1948*a*). Reports were sent by letter or telephone and opportunities for face to face consultation were, it seems, rare. Moreover, very few of the pathologists working in hospital laboratories had any special training in bacteriology.

For two conditions rather more systematic arrangements had been made, namely the venereal diseases and tuberculosis. Since 1916 local authorities had been required to make arrangements for providing practitioners with "scientific reports" on material from patients suspected of suffering from venereal disease, and by 1936 there were some 91 laboratories approved for the examination of specimens from venereal disease treatment centres and private practitioners. The Ministry's laboratory also provided some reference services. From 1913 local authorities had, in addition, been able to receive financial support for laboratory work related to the diagnosis of tuberculosis. In many cases the authorities entered into contractual arrangements with hospital or other laboratories for these tests, a situation that was to inhibit the absorption of this work, on what is essentially a communicable disease, into the ambit of the EPHLS and the PHLS.

Responsibility for the investigation of outbreaks of infection lay with the local medical officer of health, an officer of the municipal or county council. The medical officers of health had a long tradition and many of them made important contributions to our knowledge of the behaviour of infectious diseases, which formed a major element in their work. Their area of responsibility was necessarily circumscribed to the area covered by their employing authority and the only mechanism for co-ordinating investigation in different areas (apart from informal arrangements between the medical officers) lay in the hands of the small medical staff of the Ministry: the Ministry required notification of all substantial outbreaks.

The laboratory facilities for the investigation of infections and epidemics in the community were, in the years before the outbreak of war in 1939, evidently quite extensive, but they were unevenly distributed and unco-ordinated. It was recognized that they would be inadequate to cope with either of the two threats postulated as an outcome of war: firstly, bacteriological warfare, and secondly, epidemics arising from extensive population movements, from concentration in air-raid shelters, or from dislocation of water supplies, food supplies or sewage disposal. The south-east of England seemed particularly vulnerable, both from its position and from its lack even of the co-ordinating possibilities offered by the university departments in the North.

Planning for a war-time service

The problem of bacteriological warfare was first referred by the Government to a small group of bacteriologists in 1934, and in 1936 a subcommittee of the Committee on Imperial Defence was appointed under the chairmanship of Sir Maurice (later Lord) Hankey. The members of this subcommittee (the Bacteriological Warfare Subcommittee) included representatives of the Armed Forces, the Air Raid Precautions Department of the Home Office, the Chemical Defence Research Department and the Medical Research Council; three of its members were experienced medical bacteriologists. The subcommittee took a very moderate view of the possible dangers of bacteriological warfare but among the recommendations in its reports, issued in 1937 and 1938, was one on the establishment of an emergency public health laboratory service.

There is no doubt that the inspiration for the creation of such a service came from Topley. Professor W.W.C. Topley (1886–1944; Figure 1), since 1927 Professor of Bacteriology and Immunology at the London School of Hygiene and Tropical Medicine, had gained his first insight into the problems of controlling major epidemic disease when posted to Serbia, then in the throes of a typhus epidemic, in 1915. Two or three years later he started work on experimental epidemiology, using salmonella infections of mice as his model, work that was to be expanded during his tenure of the chairs of bacteriology at the University of Manchester (1922–7) and at the London School of Hygiene and Tropical Medicine. Summarizing much of the work in his Croonian Lecture in 1941, Topley wrote that, "It is quite certain that movements of susceptible and infected hosts in relation to one another, and aggregations or dispersals of human or animal herds, apart from any introduction of new infection, are sufficient to induce major changes in the incidence of many infective diseases" (Topley, 1942). This, and experience as Sheridan Delépine's successor in the Department of Bacteriology at the University of Manchester, which, as we have seen, provided public health bacteriological services for Manchester, must have been a powerful stimulus "to set himself", in the words of his obituary notice in *The Lancet* (Anon., 1944), "to make sure that . . . we should at least have an organization of bacteriologists ready and equipped to deal with the major problems of epidemic disease that might arise from air bombardment and indiscriminate evacuation [of the population from vulnerable cities]". He had become convinced that if bacteriology was to be of full service to the community it must go out into the field and make observations for itself. So, at its fifth meeting, the Bacteriological Warfare Subcommittee of the Committee on Imperial Defence received a memorandum drawn up by Professor Topley, in which he proposed "A civilian bacteriological service to operate in time of war". The subcommittee referred this memorandum to the Medical Research Council, which set up an Emergency Bacteriological Services Subcommittee, with Topley in the chair. (The full membership of this committee was as follows: W.W.C. Topley (Chairman); T. Carnwath, W.M. Scott and F. Griffith (Ministry of Health); W.W. Jameson (London School of Hygiene and Tropical Medicine); Sir Edward Mellanby and A. Landsborough Thomson (Medical Research Council); Sir John C.G. Ledingham (Lister Institute); Major H.S. Blackman (Home Office).)

After three meetings in the early months of 1938 the MRC subcommittee reported to the Bacteriological Warfare Subcommittee, whose title was changed to the Subcommittee on Emergency Bacteriological Services, with recommendations on a number of practical measures for the establishment of an Emergency Bacteriological Service. This

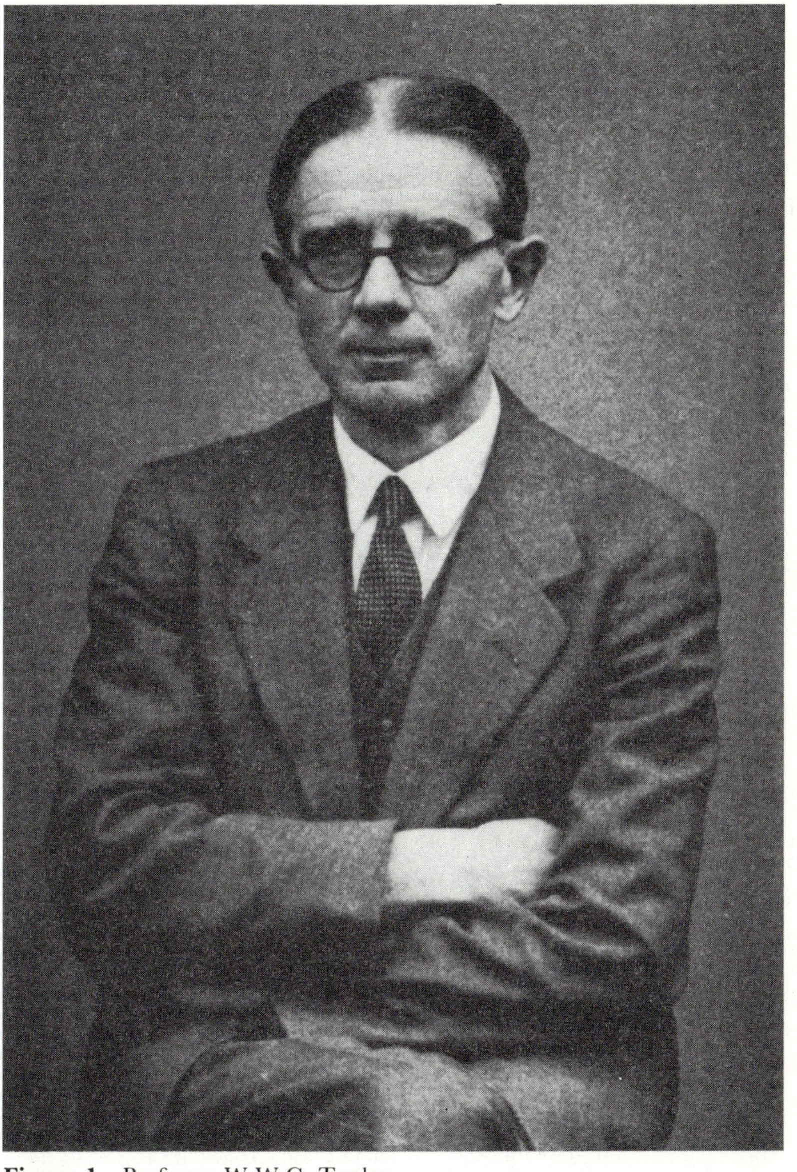

Figure 1 Professor W.W.C. Topley.

report was transmitted to the Committee on Imperial Defence on 30 June 1938.

The report recommended the establishment of a network of emergency laboratories in the southern part of England, where the provision of existing public health laboratories was weakest. The laboratories were to be staffed by workers from teaching and research institutes, particularly the London School of Hygiene and Tropical Medicine and the Ministry's Bacteriological Laboratory. (In the event, of the 13 laboratories established in the south of England and South Wales in September 1939, four were directed by individuals from the London School of Hygiene, three from the Ministry's laboratory, and the rest by individuals from various research institutes.) The new emergency laboratories were to be set up in the science departments of schools and universities, away from what were thought to be the main targets of enemy action.

The report made recommendations on the loan or purchase and storage of equipment (down to the smallest items, such as bacteriological loops), the provision of transport and of vaccines and sera, and on staffing. An indication of the distance from the present is the fact that, separate from the list of senior (all male) bacteriologists, there was a supplementary list of "some well-qualified woman bacteriologists who would be of great assistance in . . . relieving a member of the senior staff who had to leave the laboratory while carrying out a field investigation". It was not envisaged that the proposed Service would call for any central administration of a formal or continuous kind; each of the two "central laboratories" (those at Oxford and Cambridge) and many of the others would be "to a large extent autonomous". It was recognized, however, that the Medical Research Council, which, it was proposed, should be responsible for the Service, might need to set up a small committee, with representatives of the Armed Forces and appropriate Ministries, and that this committee could also provide a national intelligence centre.

The 1938 report recommended that the professors of bacteriology (or pathology) in the six universities in the North and the North Midlands (Liverpool, Manchester, Leeds, Sheffield, Birmingham and Durham (Newcastle)) should be asked to prepare local schemes for services that could be co-ordinated with the service planned for the "Southern Zone". It left the arrangements for Wales and Scotland to be determined later.

In the letter dated 20 July 1938 to Wing Commander Elliott at the office of the Committee on Imperial Defence, Sir Edward Mellanby, the Secretary of the Medical Research Council, proposed that the new service should be called the "Emergency Public Health Laboratory Service", the idea being to get rid of the word "bacteriological", which had associations in the public mind with bacteriological warfare. The Medical Research Council accepted responsibility for administering the Service on behalf of the Ministry. The achievement of this latter, seemingly surprising, arrangement certainly owes much to the persuasive powers of Dr A. (later Sir) Landsborough Thomson, who was Principal Assistant Secretary in the Medical Research Council offices and was to have administrative responsibility for the Service. Dr W. (later Sir) Wilson Jameson, at that time Professor of Public Health at the London School of Hygiene and Tropical Medicine and, from 1940, Chief Medical Officer in the Ministry of Health, was also a key figure in getting the plans accepted. The Medical Research Council further accepted responsibility, on behalf of the Ministry of Health, for running the war-time civilian blood transfusion service for London and the South-East.

Detailed planning for the new service proceeded fast during the summer and autumn of 1938; indeed the Munich crisis of September came near to calling for its mobilization. At the end of October 1938 the Ministry called a meeting of medical officers of health at which they were given full information about the organization of the planned service, the location of its laboratories and the scope of the work to be performed. The medical officers of health for the London boroughs were informed separately of the arrangements to be made for their area; originally it had been thought that the service in London could be left in the hands of the London County Council. After September 1938, however, it was decided that the Medical Research Council should take an active part and the Council set about finding suitable locations for six laboratories in the science departments of public schools in the outskirts of London. It was subsequently decided that the administration of the laboratories in the London area should be merged with the Sector administration of the Emergency Medical Services; the war-time pattern for London was to a great extent responsible for the fact that it took so long after the war for the PHLS to establish a satisfactory service in London, if indeed it has ever done so.

By mid-1939 arrangements were completed for an Emergency Public Health Laboratory Service to cover the whole of England and Wales; in Scotland it had been decided that separate arrangements should be made, based on continued reliance on university departments.

The first meeting of the prospective staff of the EPHLS laboratories was held at the London School of Hygiene and Tropical Medicine on 22 May 1939, when the plans were discussed and after which an official memorandum was issued, on 20 June. On 25 August the Medical Research Council was warned by the Ministry of the coming emergency and proceeded to transport equipment from London to Oxford; on 26 August all members of staff were told to proceed to their laboratories and by 3 September, when war was declared, most of the laboratories were fully staffed and ready for action, although it had been decreed that the equipment should not be unpacked until war had been declared. The Ministry informed medical officers of health of the establishment of the Service, which was designed "to augment existing facilities for bacteriological work required for public health purposes . . . [but] not to interfere in any way with the operation of normal services, where these could be maintained". Normal services were, of course, provided on a fee-paying basis; the EPHLS services were to be freely at the disposal of the medical officers of health (and the civil and military medical services generally) if required for the investigation and control of infectious diseases.

The Emergency Public Health Laboratory Service in War-time

Initial organization

In September 1939 there were in England and Wales a total of 19 emergency laboratories constituting the EPHLS, 13 administered by the Medical Research Council (MRC) and six associated with university departments (see Table 1 and Figure 2). Three laboratories – those at Oxford, Cambridge and Cardiff – were regarded as "central" laboratories and were headed by the medical officers from the Ministry's laboratory; Dr W.M. Scott at Oxford, Dr F. Griffith at Cambridge, and Dr V.D. Allison at Cardiff. Professor G.S. Wilson, who as Topley's close colleague at the London School of Hygiene and Tropical Medicine had played a great part in the organization of the Service, was also attached to the Oxford laboratory, which was regarded as the chief laboratory for the service as a whole, and was to act as its intelligence centre.

Dr W.M. Scott (1884–1941, Figure 3), who was in charge at Oxford, had gained his first experience in field bacteriology prior to the First World War in a study of the

Table 1 Emergency public health laboratories established in September 1939

EPHLS Southern Zone, administered by the MRC		EPHLS "associated" laboratories, attached to universities		Emergency laboratories for public health in London Sectors (EMS)	
1	Oxford (S)	14	Barnard Castle (S)	20	Brentwood (S)
2	Cambridge (U)	15	Conway (L)	21	Hertford (S)
3	Canterbury (S)	16	Kirkby Lonsdale (S)	22	Harpenden (L)
4	Gloucester (H)	17	Lincoln (L)	23	Watford (H)
5	Colchester (H)	18	Pocklington (Yorkshire) (S)	24	Ealing (H)
6	Holt (Norfolk) (S)	19	Wellington (Shropshire) (S)	25	Northwood (S)
7	Horsham (S)			26	Slough (L)
8	Sherborne (S)			27	Guildford (S)
9	Stamford (S)			28	Epsom (S)
10	Tavistock (S)			29	Downe (Kent) (L)
11	Winchester (S)				
12	Cardiff (U)				
13	Aberystwyth (L)				

The numbers refer to the map showing the location of the laboratories (Figure 2). The laboratories in the first two columns are listed in Appendix Table 1; those in the third column are given in Appendix Table 2. *Abbreviations*: U, university; S, school; H, hospital; L, laboratory in a research or other institution.

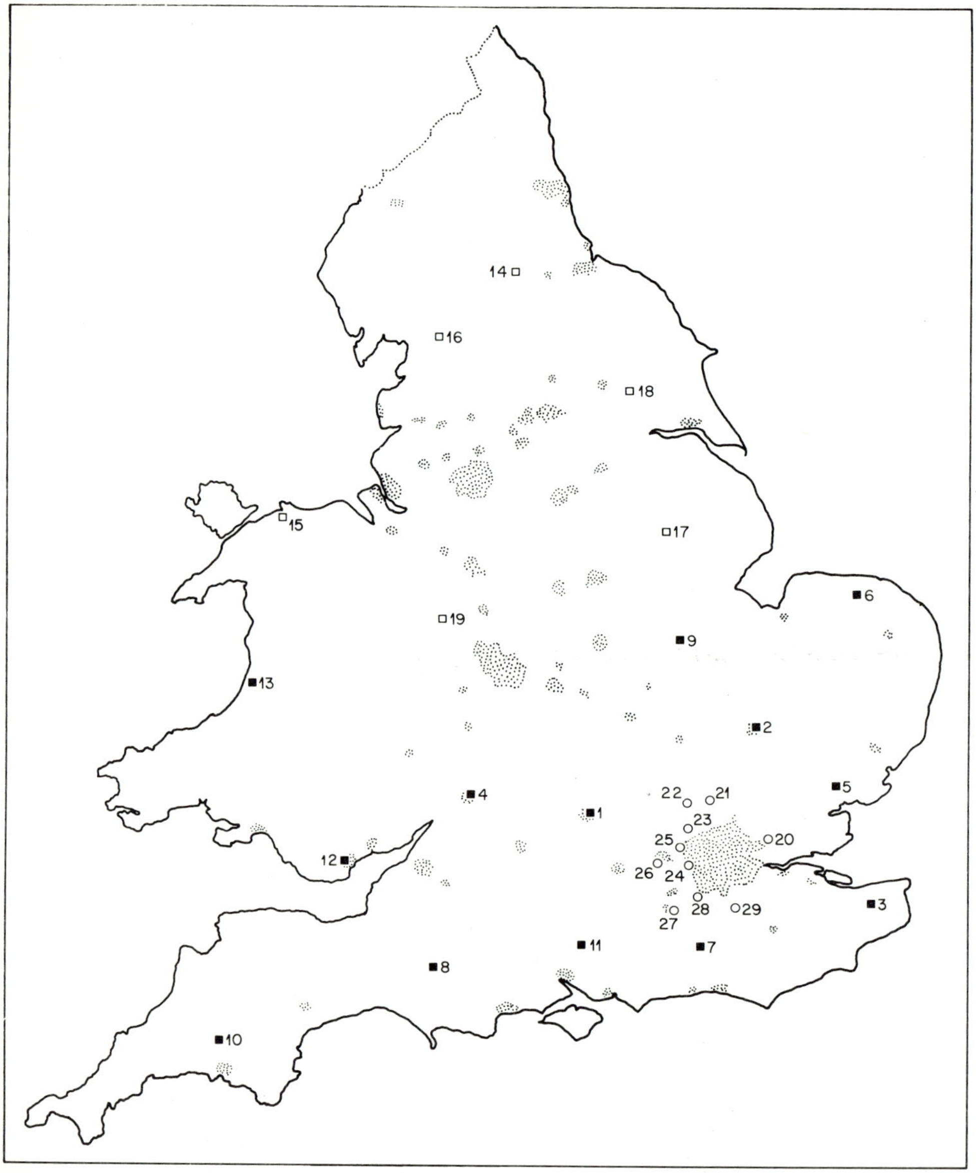

Figure 2 Emergency laboratories for public health, September 1939. ■, EPHLS laboratories administered by the MRC; □, associated laboratories administered by university departments; ○, sector public health laboratories administered by the EMS; stippling indicates main urban areas. The laboratories are listed in Table 1.

persistence of typhoid bacilli in the soil. After a short period as a medical officer of health in Kent he joined the Bacteriological Laboratory of the Local Government Board in 1917. This laboratory was taken over by the Ministry of Health in 1919. Scott developed his interest in enteric pathogens and was active in applying the serotyping schemes for salmonellas devised by Bruce White, Kauffmann and others. In the late 1930s the accounts of food-poisoning outbreaks in the Annual Reports of the Chief Medical Officer of the Ministry of Health leant heavily on Scott's work. He was also an expert on the bacteriological examination of water. Scott, and his colleague Griffith, were both dedicated bench workers and neither, it seems, was particularly attracted to administration. Both were active in the laboratory support of epidemiological investigations but they did not actually participate in the investigations in the field, a role reserved for their medical colleagues in the Ministry itself.

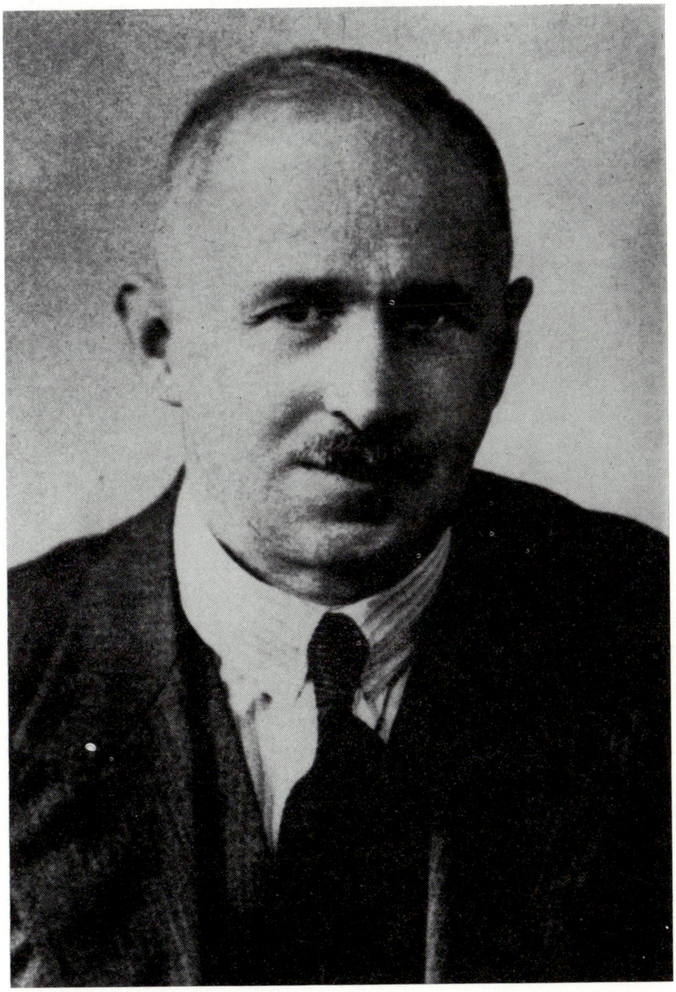

Figure 3 Dr W.M. Scott.

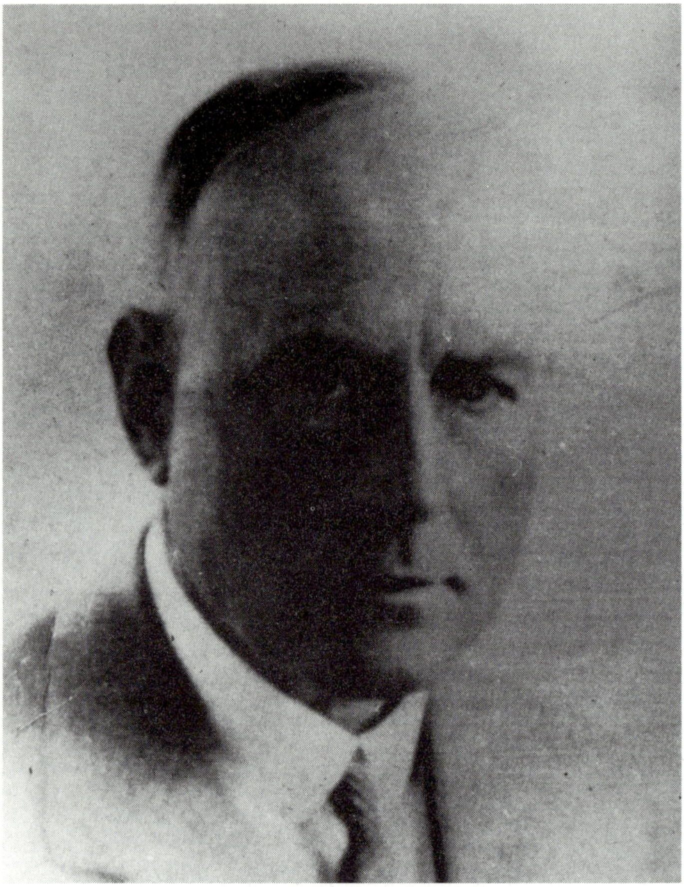

Figure 4 Dr F. Griffith.

Dr F. Griffith (1879–1941, Figure 4), who directed the Cambridge laboratory, had joined the Local Government Board (later Ministry) laboratory in 1910. Although now recognized as having, in 1928, made observations on type transformation in pneumococci that can be regarded as the earliest study in modern bacterial genetics, Griffith's main interest in the laboratory was the study of haemolytic streptococci, for which he had developed a serotyping method. With V.D. Allison and clinical colleagues this typing was applied to epidemiological studies of scarlet fever – still in the 1930s a prevalent and often serious disease – and of streptococcal infections in boarding schools. Griffith's work with Brown and Allison in scarlet fever wards had provided some of the earliest precise documentation of hospital cross-infection.

Dr V.D. Allison (1897–1982, Figure 5), directing the Cardiff laboratory, had worked with Fleming on penicillin and with J.E. McCartney in the London County Council's Southern Group Laboratory before joining the staff of the Ministry's laboratory in 1933; he had had more experience of clinical bacteriology than either

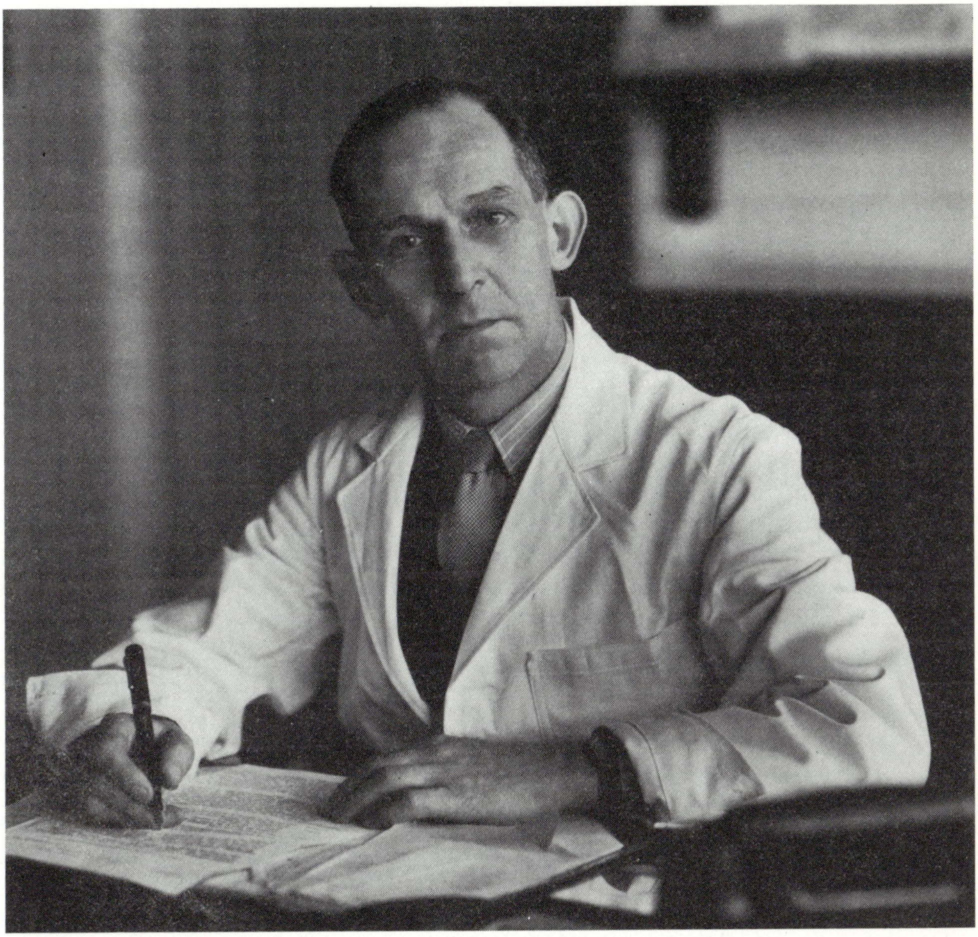

Figure 5 Dr V.D. Allison.

Scott or Griffith and he played a substantial part in the studies of cross-infection in hospitals.

The remaining 10 laboratories – those in southern England and Wales – coming directly under the administration of the MRC were mostly established in the science departments of schools. The university departments in the Midlands and the North, which in peace-time provided public health laboratory services for their areas, had established subsidiary laboratories, again mostly in schools (Table 1).

In the London area 10 emergency laboratories for public health were set up, one in each of the hospital sectors (Table 1 and Appendix Table 2), and for the duration of the war they were administered as part of the Emergency Medical Service (EMS). The senior staff of these laboratories came from the London County Council laboratories and from various hospital laboratories in the London area.

Although the university laboratories in the North and the Sector public health laboratories in London contributed epidemiological information to the EPHLS from the start, it was to be a long time before the MRC took over their administration; indeed the London laboratories all remained separate until 1946, when two of them were absorbed into the PHLS.

The staff of the emergency laboratories mostly managed to get to their designated posts by the outbreak of war. Joan Taylor recalls her arrival in Oxford and accommodation – along with Dr and Mrs Scott, Professor and Mrs Wilson and others – in fellows' rooms in the Queen's College, an event of historical importance as it was the first time such rooms had ever been designated for the use of ladies. (At that time the washing facilities in Oxford colleges were generally reached by walking across the quadrangle!) She also recalls an early picture of the Oxford laboratory with Scott and Wilson working from opposite sides of a large table – Scott's always deep in paper; Wilson's always impeccably tidy, with everything ordered before departure in the evening. But the two seem to have got on well together and Wilson had great admiration for Scott, and especially for his laboratory work; indeed Wilson has deplored the fact that so little of Scott's immense knowledge of bacteriology was committed to paper.

So the laboratories were established, but what were they to do? The Chief Medical Officer of the Ministry of Health had informed medical officers of health early in September of the existence of the emergency laboratories designed to supplement existing services. Later in the month directors of laboratories were provided with a draft letter for their local medical officer of health indicating that the laboratories could (1) examine any water supplies that were giving anxiety; (2) examine samples of milk suspected of being concerned with the spread of epidemics, or from pasteurizing plants about which there was doubt; (3) investigate cases of diphtheria, scarlet fever, tonsillitis, diarrhoea and undiagnosed pyrexia, if necessary with personal epidemiological inquiries; (4) examine material from patients with puerperal pyrexia, especially if in emergency wards. No charge was to be made and directors were encouraged to seek regular personal contact with local medical officers of health.

At the end of October 1939 a memorandum on the functions of emergency laboratories was issued from the Central Laboratory at Oxford. It recognized that, although the Service had been set up to deal with "widespread outbreaks of infectious disease occurring very soon after the outbreak of war, owing to abnormal housing conditions and general deterioration of sanitation which might be expected . . .", there had in fact been no breakdown of the general health services and infectious diseases had not been abnormally prevalent. It could, nevertheless, be anticipated that there would be winter epidemics that could be particularly difficult to control in the event of air warfare. Directors of laboratories were therefore encouraged to do all they could to bring home to medical officers of health the value of the services that the EPHLS could offer to them. It was noted that in areas already possessing good public health laboratories, the position of the new emergency laboratories was delicate, particularly if existing laboratories – or individual pathologists – had income from the examination of public health specimens. The EPHLS laboratories were to be regarded as supplementary, and were not to undertake work that could be "capably" provided by existing laboratories, but there was the rider that a "necessity exists nearly everywhere normally – and still more in war-time – for a great increase in public health bacteriological work if the [medical officer of health] is to be kept properly informed . . .". There was, moreover, an opportunity for epidemiological research, "particularly into the distribution of infective agents resulting from war-time changes . . .". Any opportunity for observation of outbreaks of enteritis, or of respiratory infections in semi-closed communities, should be seized for intensive work.

Dyke (1961) has commented that Topley, having been nurtured in academic institutes, seemed initially to have been "naively unaware" of the part already being played by the pathology services of the provincial, non-teaching, voluntary hospitals. But he had soon realized the value of these resources, as is evident from the number of hospital laboratories given the title of Associated Laboratory during 1940 (see below and Appendix Table 3).

The EPHLS was essentially a bacteriological service, for the control of communicable diseases. During the war years it had a small Chemical Reference Laboratory under Professor M.E. Delafield, but chemical analyses for public health purposes never became a routine function of the Service and they have continued to the present to be provided by the largely independent public analysts, with some support from the Laboratory of the Government Chemist.

During the war years there was also a Bacterial Sabotage Reference Laboratory, directed by Dr P. Bruce White, which examined a great variety of "suspicious objects", none of which, in fact, proved to be of enemy origin.

The Director of the Service

The papers circulated from the Central Laboratory at Oxford were unsigned; there was at the time no officially designated Director of the EPHLS. According to Thomson (1975), W.M. Scott, of the Ministry of Health Laboratory, was made Director of the Service. Wilson, in his "Historical notes . . .", referring to the administration of the Service at the time, writes that he does not think that Scott had the title of Director, and doubts whether he would have wished it, partly because his colleague, Griffith, was senior in years of experience. Wilson records that major decisions were taken by Thomson, Topley, Scott and Wilson in collaboration. Scott was certainly regarded as the Director of the Oxford laboratory, although he actually left much of the administration to Wilson, and, as *de facto* administrative head of the Ministry's laboratory, would certainly have been regarded as the appropriate person to direct the EPHLS. Yet the inspiration for the Service undoubtedly stemmed from Topley; he was attached to the MRC head office as technical adviser on the Service and should probably be regarded as the main source of leadership in the early months. The Advisory Committee postulated in the original Committee on Imperial Defence paper was never set up. Topley is reported to have disbanded many advisory committees when he moved to the Agricultural Research Council, and the pattern of "personal" administration of the Service was to persist for many years in the partnership of Wilson and Thomson.

Scott had returned to London from Oxford in April 1940 and had a laboratory at the London School of Hygiene and Tropical Medicine, where the offices of the MRC and of the EPHLS were situated, and early in 1941 he was promoted to Senior Medical

Officer and designated head of the Ministry's Laboratory Division. The Report of the Chief Medical Officer records that he was formally designated Director of the EPHLS. Very shortly afterwards, he was killed in an air-raid on London during the night of 16/17 April. Wilson, again in his "Historical notes . . .", remarks that the Service "had become well established . . . when its first Director died . . .".

Topley had already been appointed to the post of Secretary to the Agricultural Research Council and took up his duties there on 28 April 1941. And so, not long after Scott's death, G.S. Wilson was formally appointed Director of the EPHLS.

G.S. Wilson (*b.* 1895, Frontispiece) – "G.S." to the world at large – had worked with Topley at Charing Cross Hospital and went with him to Manchester where his principal research interests, into the bacteriological control of milk and brucellosis, were started. These were stimulated by the extensive public health practice enjoyed by the University Department of Bacteriology, an inheritance from its founder, Sheridan Delépine. The Manchester years saw the production of the first edition of the world-famous bacteriologists' bible: Topley and Wilson's *Principles of Bacteriology and Immunity*. Wilson moved with Topley to the newly founded London School of Hygiene and Tropical Medicine in 1927 and not only continued his own work on milk, but also collaborated with Topley in his work on the epidemiology of salmonella and ectromelia infections in colonies of mice. Wilson had been intimately concerned with pre-war planning of the EPHLS and in the administration of the Service when it started. He and A. Landsborough Thomson, the Principal Assistant Secretary in the MRC who then – and for long afterwards – was untiring in his work for the Service, had great mutual respect for one another, so that when Topley left to go to the Agricultural Research Council, and Scott was killed, the appointment of Wilson as Director ensured continuity of thought and development. Like Topley, Wilson was no great believer in committee administration and from 1941 until he retired in 1963, the direction and administration of the EPHLS and subsequently of the PHLS might almost be described as "Wilson and Thomson Limited". Wilson has said that much of what he did was what Topley had planned, but there can be no possible doubt that the success of the Service, and the status that it has achieved in Britain and in the world beyond, is in large part attributable to Wilson's leadership and, in particular, to his determination that the work of the Service should always be of the highest scientific standards.

Charges for services

The original Ministry memorandum at the outbreak of war made it clear that the services of the emergency laboratories were available to the civil and military health authorities for help in the control of infectious disease, without charge. The MRC was reimbursed for the cost of the Service from Ministry funds. Subsequently, when it became clear that the laboratories had not experienced the envisaged emergency calls, but that they were actively participating in laboratory work on behalf of local health authorities, the Ministry felt that such work should be paid for by the authorities. The MRC resisted any suggestion of a "fee per specimen" charge, on the grounds that it would inhibit the full use of the laboratories, which it was desirable to encourage. Eventually a compromise was reached by which local authorities reimbursed the MRC with a block grant at a rate equivalent to the sum the authority had spent on laboratory services before the war. In return the EPHLS was prepared to give unlimited service within an agreed schedule. This proved satisfactory to the local authorities, and indeed many of them discarded their peace-time arrangements and transferred all their work to the emergency laboratories. By 1941 these block grant arrangements had been agreed by 17 counties, three county boroughs, 97 urban districts and municipal boroughs, 71 rural districts and seven joint hospital boards. There was, not unnaturally, considerable resentment in some quarters at the intrusion of the free service into an area that had previously offered a source of legitimate earnings to a number of individuals and hospitals. This enmity persisted in one form or another for many years, though after the establishment of the "free" National Health Service the basis of the enmity was changed.

Associated laboratories

As the situation developed the laboratories established by the universities in the Midlands and the North developed a formalized relation with the EPHLS as "Associated Laboratories". They reported to EPHLS headquarters on their activities and on any findings that proved the existence of serious infectious disease; they also agreed to provide a service similar to that offered by the EPHLS laboratories themselves. In 1940 and subsequently a number of hospital laboratories that were already providing public health bacteriological services joined the list of associated laboratories under the same terms. For convenience, Appendix Table 3 lists all the laboratories accorded "associated" status from 1939 to the end of 1958, when the last of them, Bristol, became a constituent laboratory.

The relation of the associated laboratories to the rest of the Service seems to have been pretty much an arm's length affair; Cayton, who directed the last laboratory to transfer from "associated" to constituent status, recalled that few opportunities were offered for active scientific participation in the affairs of the Service.

The Monthly Bulletin

The *Monthly Bulletin of the Emergency Public Health Laboratory Service* had its origin in cyclostyled notes circulated to the laboratories from a very early stage in the development of the Service: the first issue of a monthly "progress report" appeared in November 1939 (and an early issue includes among other matters hints on the use of discarded culture media as a garden fertilizer). The bulletin appeared in printed form from November 1941. The brief epidemiological reports included in it were usually reprinted in the *Bulletin of Hygiene* and so reached a wide audience in the public health field; it also carried notes on various laboratory techniques. From 1943 the bulletin incorporated a section from the Ministry and was known as the *Monthly Bulletin of the Ministry of Health and Emergency Public Health Laboratory Service*, and its value as a vehicle for important epidemiological investigations is demonstrated by the considerable number of papers from it that I have cited in this account. The laboratory section was edited for many years by Wilson himself, in his usual meticulous manner, and assisted by his secretary, Miss Madeleine Barry.

The Monthly Bulletin continued publication until 1967, the editing of the laboratory section latterly being in the hands of J.C. Kelsey; in 1967 the Department of Health and Social Security, as it had by then become, decided that its contribution deserved a glossier publication, known as *Health Trends*, and the laboratory section disappeared.

Scientific Work of the Emergency Public Health Laboratory Service

Public health bacteriology in the pre-war years had consisted very largely of the examination of throat swabs for diphtheria bacilli and to a less extent haemolytic streptococci, and of faeces for enteric pathogens, together with serological tests for enteric fever and tests on the sanitary quality of milk and water. The report of the Chief Medical Officer of the Ministry of the war years stated that the active participation of the emergency laboratories in the investigation of outbreaks of diphtheria, dysentery, scarlet fever and the like was one of the most fruitful developments of public health practice. These field investigations were always conducted at the request, or with the consent of, the local medical officer of health and "for the first time it was possible to apply methods of modern bacteriology and immunology in the field, unhampered by considerations of cost".

In a report to the Medical Research Council in December 1941, Wilson recorded that the Army had been quick to recognize the potential advantages of the emergency laboratories and had made good use of them. The reaction of the medical officers of health had been variable, some because they already had their own facilities, some because they were quite unused to seeking bacteriological help. The laboratory directors had had to make the medical officers of health understand the inadequacies of their arrangements, and impress on them what could be provided. This had all taken time, and without the research projects developed in the early months of the war, some of the laboratories would have been practically idle.

The growth of the work of the laboratories is illustrated by the following figures for numbers of specimens examined in four-week periods:

to 28 October 1939,	929;
to 25 November 1939,	1,705;
to 29 October 1940,	20,289;
to 31 December 1941,	247,214.

Diphtheria

One major success story was that of diphtheria, still a very prevalent infection: in 1941 the 20 laboratories isolated *Corynebacterium diphtheriae* from no fewer than 8457 cases or convalescents and even in 1944 there were nearly 6000 such isolations. Very soon after commencing work in 1939, a number of laboratories became involved in investigating small outbreaks in schools and in exploring the use of combined active–passive immunization, together with the detection and exclusion of carriers, for the control of such outbreaks. Indeed, in the report describing the method (Fulton *et al.*, 1941), two of the outbreaks had been studied in December 1939, a good indication of the rapidity with which the Oxford laboratory established collaborative working arrangements with the local medical officers of health. At the same time several EPHLS laboratories collaborated in volunteer studies on the effect of combining active and passive immunization. Collaborative studies were also soon under way for improving the laboratory diagnosis of diphtheria – Hoyle's tellurite medium (Hoyle, 1941) had been tested in three laboratories – and several other studies of cultural methods were reported by Knox (1944).

The Ministry of Health initiated a mass vaccination programme with diphtheria toxoid at the end of 1940 and EPHLS laboratories took part in a number of trials of different makes of toxoid: early studies revealed substantial differences between toxoids

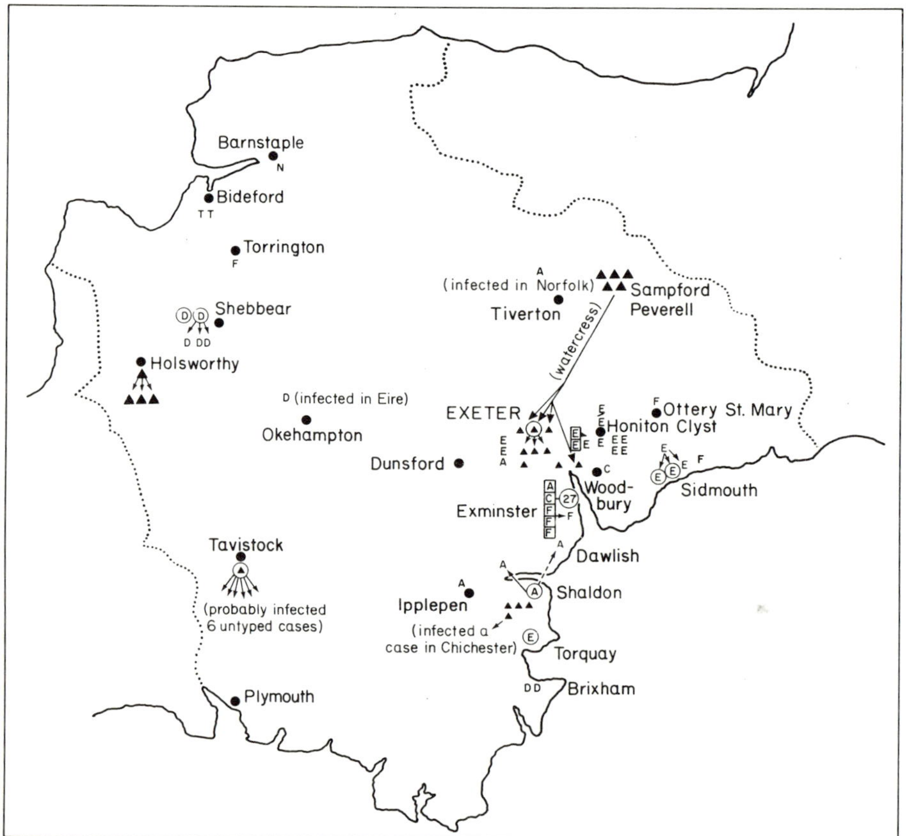

Figure 6 Distribution of typhoid cases and carriers in Devon, 1941–4. *Note*: a letter within a circle denotes a chronic carrier of that type; a letter within a square denotes a chronic carrier in a mental hospital. Vi types: A, type A; C, type C; D, type D1; E, type E1; F, type F1; ▲, type 91; T, untypable; N, new type "Richmond". The symbol ㉗ indicates a type C outbreak of 27 cases. (Redrawn after Cruickshank, 1947.)

that led to a tightening of the manufacturing specifications. Indeed studies of diphtheria prophylactics were to be a recurrent topic of research for several years after the war ended. By 1944 nearly 5.5 million children had been vaccinated and the annual number of deaths had declined to 934, from the 1940 figure of 2480.

Enteric fever

In 1939 there were more than 1500 notifications of enteric fever and during the war years the laboratories investigated a considerable number of outbreaks, mostly small. The wide provision, through the EPHLS, of serological and cultural diagnostic facilities enabled the Ministry to require separate notification of typhoid and paratyphoid fever from July 1941. Dr A. Felix had developed the phage typing scheme devised by Craigie and Yen, which provided a method for "finger-printing" typhoid bacilli, and he joined the EPHLS to form an Enteric Reference Laboratory, located first at Oxford and subsequently successively at the London School of Hygiene and Tropical Medicine, the Wellcome Research Institute, and the National Institute for Medical Research. A phage typing service was made available to EPHLS and other laboratories from 1940 and Felix went on to develop a scheme for *Salmonella paratyphi* B. In 1943 he was able to describe the use of phage typing in some 440 cases of typhoid fever occurring in a considerable number of small outbreaks, and Bradley (1943) was able, with the help of Felix's laboratory, to track to one original source no fewer than 23 infections occurring in five different counties. Cruickshank (1947) used the typing method to elucidate the relation between cases of typhoid fever – 83 in number – occurring in Devon during 1941–4 (Figure 6).

Felix (1941) was also responsible for the introduction of the alcohol-killed typhoid vaccine, postulated to be a better immunogen on the basis of experimental work, largely in mice and rabbits. It was not until the alcohol-killed preparation was compared with the more conventional acetone-killed vaccine in a field trial in man (Yugoslav Typhoid Commission, 1962) that the fallacy of relying on the animal tests was recognized.

Food poisoning

There was striking increase in the number of food-poisoning outbreaks reported to the Ministry during the war years, doubtless attributable both to the increase in diagnostic facilities and to the great increase in communal feeding. In the Ministry's laboratory, Scott had been active in the 1930s in applying modern serotyping methods for salmonellas to strains isolated from food-poisoning incidents. He continued this while at Oxford, and after he left Oxford in 1940 the work was taken over by Joan Taylor. Reports of salmonella food poisoning increased dramatically, from around 100 in 1942 to over 450 in 1944. While most of the strains fell into serotypes well known as the cause of food poisoning in Britain, no fewer than 10 serotypes new to Britain were recognized in 1942, a further eight in 1943 and six in 1944. These serotypes were also found among the salmonellas isolated from the dried-egg powder imported from the United States as a valuable source of protein, and first distributed to the public in July 1942. Moreover the serotypes were among those known to be present in chicken flocks in the United States. There seems no doubt that part at least of this rise in salmonella food poisoning could be attributed to consumption of dried egg, contaminated by salmonellas at source and not adequately cooked before consumption (MRC, 1947). This work demonstrated well the benefits flowing from a national network of laboratories supported by a reference service able to make precise identification and to assemble the epidemiological information. At the time the EPHLS did not have any staff identified as "epidemiologists", although Scott had tried to persuade the Ministry of the need for such workers. But the laboratory directors, albeit trained as bacteriologists, were in many cases keen to take an active part in the field epidemiological investigations and were encouraged to do so both by the MRC – in the persons doubtless of Topley and later Wilson – and in many cases by the local medical officers of health.

As a supplement to the elucidation of the role of dried egg in the etiology of food poisoning, a number of EPHLS laboratories examined mesenteric lymph nodes from about 5000 pigs for the presence of salmonellas, since it was known that some of the imported dried egg was used as animal feedstuff; 10 serotypes were identified, similar to those from food-poisoning cases, which had never previously been found in Britain and were almost certainly derived from the dried egg.

Although food poisoning that must have been due to the enterotoxin of *Staphylococcus aureus* was first described at the end of the last century, it was not until the 1930s that it was commonly recognized. But it is striking that of some 296 outbreaks of food poisoning investigated by the Ministry's officers during the war years, 115 were of the "toxin type". The EPHLS laboratories were involved in many studies, and a number of outbreaks in Oxford at Easter 1945 afforded an early indication of the value of phage typing of staphylococci for tracking the source of infection.

Fulton, also working at Oxford, studied the staphylococcal enterotoxin, and its detection by the kitten test.

Dysentery

Dysentery notifications also increased steadily during the war years, but in this case laboratory investigations, while documenting the increase, were not able to offer a solution to the problem of control.

Staphylococcal infections

For the most part the work of the emergency laboratories was carried out on behalf of medical officers of health and general practitioners on material from patients in the community or, in some cases, in infectious diseases hospitals. However, Allison and Hobbs, in Cardiff, and the directors of several other laboratories, investigated staphylococcal infections in maternity homes. The developing interest in staphylococcal infections in hospitals, of which the Cardiff work was one example but which was mostly concentrated outside the EPHLS, nevertheless stimulated work in the Service on the development of typing techniques for staphylococci. Betty Hobbs tried hard to develop a usable method from Cowan's serological analysis, while Wilson and

Atkinson (1945), at Oxford, successfully developed a method of phage typing that was to be of immense value in the studies of the hospital staphylococcal pandemic of the 1950s and 1960s, and which undoubtedly helped to interest the PHLS in infections spreading within hospitals as well as those spreading in the community.

Whooping cough

Whooping cough was, like diphtheria, a substantial killing disease in the 1940s. Following some American work indicating that a bacterial vaccine could induce protective immunity, McFarlan and colleagues carried out small field trials in 1942–4 (McFarlan *et al.*, 1945); these did not support the earlier American view but the subject was recognized to be of such importance that it was taken up again very soon after the end of the war in much more substantial – and encouraging – trials (see p. 66).

Other infections

There was very little scope for diagnostic virology in the early 1940s but the EPHLS was able to participate in studies to determine the prevalence of antibodies to the influenza virus in the population. The MRC organized epidemiological studies of hepatitis, to which the EPHLS contributed, but, in the absence of precise diagnostic methods, could not do much more.

The war years saw two epidemics in which EPHLS laboratories were not notably concerned, namely the outbreak of meningococcal meningitis in 1939–41 (although several laboratories collaborated in surveys of the carrier state), and the rise in the incidence of syphilis and gonorrhoea which lasted until the late 1940s. The explanation for the lack of interest in the latter is that, as already mentioned, laboratory facilities for the study of venereal diseases had been developed quite systematically before the war and the Ministry supported a small reference laboratory (later transferred to the PHLS as the Venereal Diseases Reference Laboratory) which was principally concerned with the preparation of standard reagents. For similar reasons EPHLS laboratories were not greatly concerned with tuberculosis in man, though they tested milks for tubercle bacilli and several participated in an extensive field study of the frequency of bovine tubercle bacilli in patients with non-pulmonary tuberculosis (PHLS 1949*a*). A.Q. Wells, at Oxford, worked on the vole tubercle bacillus as a possible immunizing agent and some work was also carried out on cultivation of bacilli from laryngeal swabs.

Administrative Development

During the war years, as the effect (or lack of effect) of enemy action on infectious diseases became apparent, and as the potential benefits of a national system of public health laboratories were appreciated, changes were made in the location and staffing of the laboratories (Appendix Table 1). Most of the laboratories originally established in schools were closed, or in some cases transferred to County Council laboratories which were taken over by the Service; in other cases accommodation was found in hospitals. Five new laboratories were opened, all but one on hospital premises.

The very fact that the emergency laboratories did not have to deal with unusual bacteriological problems – as had been feared – meant that they were able to contribute their expertise to the study of infectious diseases then "normally" prevalent in the country and in doing so demonstrate the great benefit that could flow from a nationally organized laboratory service. The weekly reporting of pertinent laboratory findings to the EPHLS headquarters provided information on the prevalence of many infections to an extent otherwise unobtainable. The regular interchange of information between laboratories facilitated the introduction of new laboratory and epidemiological methods, as well as providing excellent opportunities for research in which groups of laboratories participated. And the fact that, from the first, the laboratories had been encouraged to undertake epidemiological investigations demonstrated that the provision of an integrated laboratory service could add a significant new dimension to the medical officer of health's capacity to unravel problems in the control of infectious diseases.

It is interesting to note that the MRC committee reporting to the government in 1938 on the need for an emergency bacteriological service had written:

> "Although the organization of the public health laboratory services in peace-time does not fall within our terms of reference, we would wish to express the opinion that the existing position is extremely unsatisfactory and to point out that the provision of an adequate and integrated national public health laboratory service . . . would not only improve the co-ordination of public health laboratory work in the country, bringing it to a level already obtained in many countries in Europe and the United States . . ."

By 1944 these advantages had been demonstrated in practice and the stage was set for the planning of a permanent service.

The EPHLS had been established to investigate and control infectious diseases, and the planning of the permanent Service adhered to this concept; so far as I am aware there was no extended discussion of the possibility of creating a Service that would provide laboratory support for the public health services in the fields, for example, of environmental pollution or toxicology.

Plans for a permanent PHLS

In the discussions that eventually led to the agreement to establish a permanent service, Wilson, Dr Philip Panton, the Ministry's adviser on pathology, and Professor S.P. Bedson advocated a single national laboratory service, containing one division for hospital pathology and one for public health bacteriology. It was accepted that epidemiological considerations ruled out the practicability of administering a public health laboratory service on the regional basis that was planned for the hospital service. However, the Ministry's officers considered that it would not be administratively satisfactory to impose a nationally administered laboratory service on a regionally administered hospital service, and, with the benefit of 40 years' hindsight, it seems clear that they were right. The burgeoning of the hospital pathological services generally and the extent to which the medical staff of the laboratories are concerned with day to day management of patients, makes it virtually essential that the senior staff of the laboratory should be seen by their clinical colleagues to be fully a part of the hospital staff. The development of joint hospital/public health laboratories, which will be discussed later, has certainly provided a mechanism by which a nationally administered service can participate fully in hospital work, but a system that works (albeit not without difficulties) for some 50–60 laboratories is not necessarily a good model for one comprising about 400 laboratories.

At all events, the decision was made to incorporate into the 1944 White Paper on the National Health Service, the proposal to establish a separate national Public Health Laboratory Service to cover England and Wales, and in April 1944 the Chief Medical Officer, Sir Wilson Jameson, wrote to the Secretary of the Medical Research Council, Sir Edward Mellanby, expressing the hope that the Council would continue to administer the Service, at least for a few years. It was proposed that, starting from the nucleus comprised by the EPHLS, the new service would expand gradually, and ultimately consist of a central laboratory in London, 10 regional laboratories at university centres in England and Wales, and possibly some 60 smaller local laboratories. The figure of 70 for the total number of laboratories seems to have been "an informed guess" (or "plucked out of the air"). Wilson has said that, as far as he could recall, there was no detailed plan to justify this number; and Sir George Godber has confirmed this in a letter to me. The annual cost, to be borne by the Exchequer, was estimated at about £400,000 when the Service was fully operational, and this was not expected for several years.

It was argued that the MRC was the appropriate body to manage the Service for several reasons: the Service could act as a training ground in laboratory methods and as a "selective filter" for recruits to pure research; it could perform a valuable function in throwing up problems for fundamental research; and it would be able to carry out field trials in extension of the work of research institutes. Moreover, it was said that only the MRC could provide the scientific support and guidance needed for the practical application of bacteriological methods to epidemiological problems, which would itself constitute a major research topic. In more detailed proposals considered by the Council at its June 1944 meeting, it was made clear that, while the MRC would have full administrative and technical control of the Service, and the staff would be its employees, it would have to consult the Ministry on questions of policy such as enlarging the scope of the work, location of laboratories, salary scales and some other matters. The Council would be provided with earmarked funds from the Ministry of Health Vote (the MRC at that time coming under the Privy Council).

The members of the Medical Research Council were, not surprisingly, divided on the wisdom of taking on the administration of a peace-time routine service, which might interfere with their proper research activities, and they asked for details of the Service's research programme, and of the administrative requirements.

In response it was stated that all the routine administrative functions would be undertaken by the Director and heads of laboratories and that, at the time, the headquarters administration of the EPHLS called for a very small staff. In fact, as Wilson wrote in his "Historical notes . . .", the whole tone of the memorandum was to play down the magnitude of the administrative burden that the Council would have to bear.

The memorandum on the research programme opened with a statement of the training programme for medical staff, which it was implied might provide useful recruits for the MRC. The research topics envisaged included improved methods of diagnosis; routine surveys of the type distribution of prevalent organisms; studies of the mode of spread of certain diseases and methods for forecasting and controlling epidemics; and trials of prophylactic and therapeutic agents. The memorandum also indicated that the reference laboratories would undertake "fundamental" research on pathogenic bacteria, and the application of the results of that research to epidemiology.

The Council was persuaded by these two memoranda, and, doubtless, by the advocacy of Landsborough Thomson. Mellanby, in seeking the agreement of the Lord President of the Privy Council, to whom the MRC was accountable, laid great stress on the research activities of the Service and on the probability that the Service would deteriorate or collapse unless the qualified staff were assured that they would be under the control (*sic* – the consultative era was still a long way off) of the Medical Research Council and not some other body. This last argument may have had some validity, for the war-time service had established a strong *esprit de corps* and staff had great respect for the liberal administrative traditions of the MRC. And, without doubt, the carry-over of these traditions to the post-war PHLS was of immense value. The device of persuading the MRC to administer what was essentially to be a routine service did, however, have penalties that were to become obvious before long, and the equivocal relation of the PHLS to the rest of the National Health Service, stemming from this device, continues to generate serious problems to this day. The postulated reciprocal benefit for the PHLS and the MRC in respect of research cannot really be said to have materialized in the way that one might suppose the persuasive memorandum was designed to imply. Although several members of the PHLS staff went on to become successful research workers with the MRC, and the Council called on the PHLS to provide an organizational base for some of its field trials of immunizing agents, there were relatively few collaborative projects with MRC staff, perhaps in large part because the MRC's interests in the 1950s were directed more to "basic" than to "applied" research.

By September 1944 agreement had been reached and the formal decision that the MRC should have administrative responsibility for the peace-time Service, for an initial period of five years, was conveyed to the Council at its meeting on 22 September.

During the war years, the public health bacteriology for Scotland was provided largely by the laboratories in the four Scottish universities; although the National Health Service was to cover Scotland, it was not proposed that the PHLS should be expanded to cover Scotland. Suggestions were made from time to time over the years for development of formal links, but none proved acceptable.

A paper prepared for the Ministry by L. Banks and George Godber (later Chief Medical Officer) in the summer of 1944 had proposed the establishment of a hierarchical network of "area" laboratories, each serving a population of 0.5–1 million, each under a regional laboratory in a university centre that would give supervision and support. All public health bacteriology should be carried out in these special laboratories, except in areas too remote from them, where "associated" hospital laboratories might do some public health work. In September 1944 Wilson outlined the proposed structure of the new service very much along the same lines. His statement emphasized the need for the Service to be satisfied with the methods used in associated laboratories, and the need to receive duplicate reports on the public health work done in them. It was thought that, in some hospitals, it might be economical for the public health laboratory to undertake all the bacteriological work, although only that in connection with infectious diseases would be free of charge.

A draft memorandum along these lines was submitted to a meeting of heads of constituent EPHLS laboratories in October 1944. From the record it appears that the meeting became somewhat bogged down in minutiae, as there were several follow-up letters from directors. Allison wrote a percipient note in which he stressed the need for public health bacteriologists to maintain some clinical contacts – and the fever hospital was the only place open to them to do it; he felt that tuberculosis and venereal diseases should come within the terms of reference of the PHLS, and he recognized the scope for conflict with the sanitary inspectors, who were the "epidemic officers" in some areas, with the public analysts, and with local authorities that had a financial interest in public health bacteriology.

Charges for services

There was also much discussion on the question of which, if any, laboratory examinations should attract fees. Wilson was determined that all examinations made for the diagnosis, control or prevention of infectious diseases should be free from all charges, but felt that the "free service should not include examinations carried out for the diagnosis of non-infectious disease, or of infective diseases unlikely to be of public health importance". Wilson's notes do not mention examinations used for the control of treatment – the antibiotic era was only just dawning – and they clearly equate "public health importance" with communicability in the general population. It was fortunate that, before long, the introduction of the totally free National Health Service

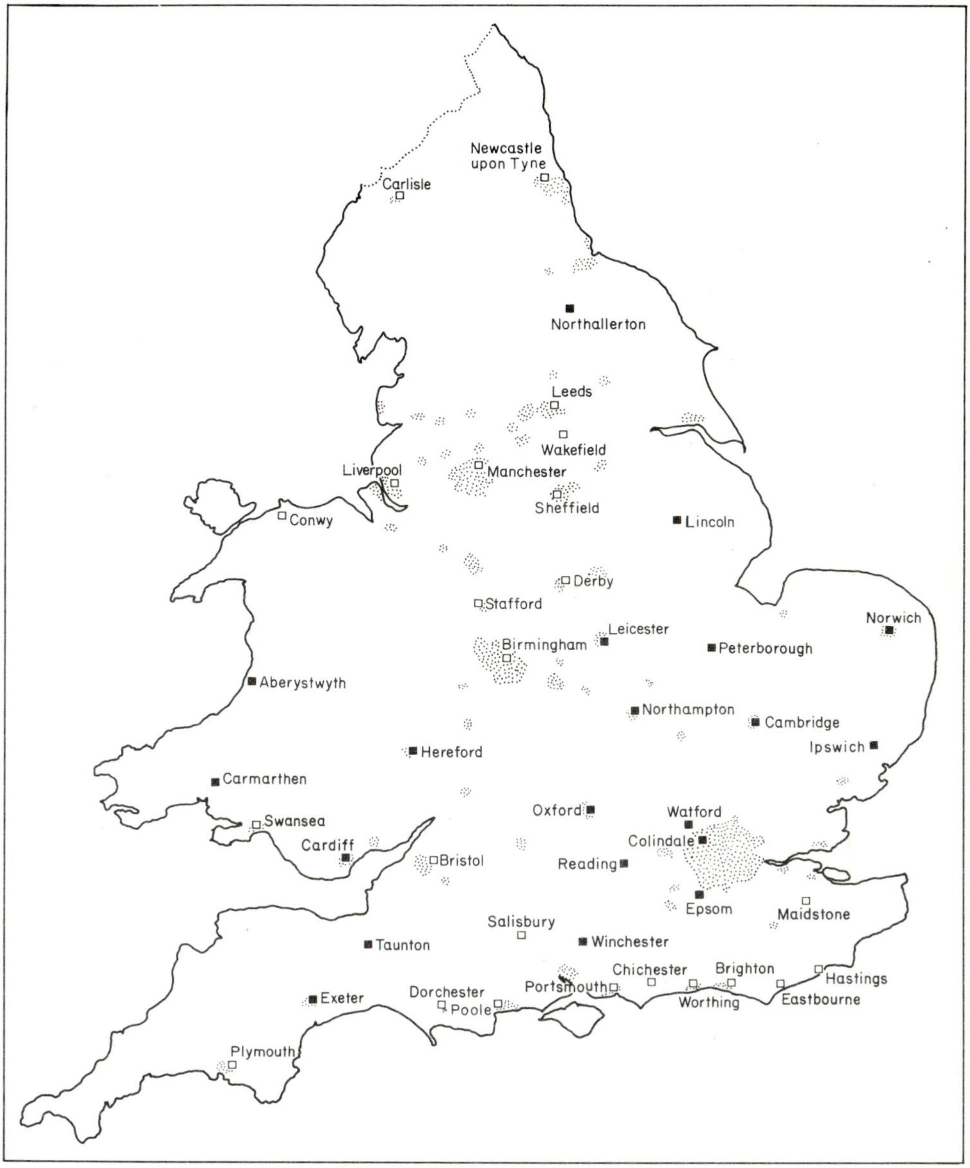

Figure 7 PHLS laboratories, December 1946. ■, area/regional PHLS laboratories; □, associated laboratories.

made the somewhat metaphysical distinction of "public health importance" redundant.

Tuberculosis and venereal diseases raised problems because, as noted earlier, there was in existence a fairly general service that was a source of income to individuals or institutions. So it was decided that the free service should not extend to the examination of material for tubercle bacilli nor for the agents of venereal disease, except in the case of patients "in whom a diagnosis had not yet been reached, who were still at large, and who, before being brought under treatment . . . constituted a menace to the public health". On further consideration, the exemption from charging for some tests for venereal diseases was deleted; all were to be charged.

Similar complications arose over the examination of milk; while tests made in relation to suspected milk-borne disease, and those on "consumer" milks submitted by sanitary inspectors, were to be free, those tests for cleanliness, or for tubercle bacilli or brucellae submitted by producers, would be charged for.

An important decision reached at this time was that the reference laboratories, which were already in embryo and which it was planned to expand substantially (to carry out type identification and other special tests outside the range of a diagnostic laboratory), should be available to assist all laboratories throughout the country, without charge. Not only did this save an immense amount of book-keeping and argument, e.g. as to who should pay any fee, but it provided a valuable link between the PHLS and the developing hospital bacteriological services at a time when so few of the area laboratories were in hospitals.

The eventual National Health Service Act, which received Royal Assent on 6 November 1946, empowered the Minister of Health "to provide a bacteriological service . . . for the control of the spread of infectious diseases" and the preparations were so far advanced that the Public Health Laboratory Service – no longer Emergency – came into being immediately, although the implementation of the free service had to wait until the start of the new financial year on 1 April 1947.

The laboratories in operation at 6 November 1946 are shown in Figure 7. There were 19 "constituent laboratories", the laboratories of the EPHLS plus the Routine Diagnostic Laboratory at Colindale, and 27 "associated laboratories", many of which would subsequently become constituent laboratories (Appendix Table 3). After the permanent PHLS came into existence in 1946 those associated laboratories not incorporated into the Service received a subsidy from central funds to enable them to provide free services similar to those provided by the PHLS laboratories. All had ceased to be "associated", for one reason or another, by the end of 1958.

It was decided early in the planning of the post-war Service that the reference laboratories should, as far as was practicable, be brought together into one central laboratory, and it was fortunate that suitable premises became available when the Ministry decided that the production of smallpox vaccine at the Government Lymph Establishment at Colindale in North London should cease.

The Public Health Laboratory Service: the First Decade

An account of the evolution of the PHLS from the point at which the decision had been made to set it up on a permanent basis has to review both its administrative development and its scientific work. For convenience, the 35-year period from 1946 to 1980 has been divided into three phases: 1946–56, 1957–69, and 1970–80.

The decade from 1946 saw the end of smallpox as a regular annual entry in the public health statistics, the decline in diphtheria from 12,000 cases a year to fewer than 100, and of enteric fever from 500 to little over 100; it also saw the greatest ever epidemic of poliomyelitis, the rise and fall of an epidemic of infantile diarrhoea, a sevenfold rise in reported food poisoning and a sevenfold rise in reported dysentery. Furthermore, though nowhere appearing in the national statistics, the decade saw the epidemic of infections due to antibiotic-resistant bacteria in hospitals.

During the same decade, the PHLS grew from 21 laboratories to 57, in large part by the incorporation of associated laboratories that were already providing public health bacteriological services, and it established 10 reference and special laboratories, eight of them in the Central Public Health Laboratory at Colindale. An early policy decision determined that the laboratories ought to be sited on hospital premises, a decision that was inevitably to determine that the Service would become orientated to clinical microbiology and so divorced from the non-microbiological aspects of public health. Nor would it develop along the lines, originally devised by Robert Koch and still operating in several of the Eastern European countries, of a network of "sanitary/epidemiological stations". At the start the Service was purely a community-orientated public health laboratory service, only three of the laboratories carrying out routine general hospital bacteriology. By 1956, 20 of the 57 laboratories were acting as hospital bacteriological laboratories as well as carrying on their public health functions; just half of the laboratories incorporated in the PHLS between 1946 and 1956 were in hospitals (see Figure 24, p. 85). After 1956 only one of the new laboratories (Bristol) was established outside a hospital.

The laboratory network

The "master plan" (cf. p. 26, above) for the development of the PHLS, agreed between the MRC and the Ministry, was for a network of about 70 laboratories distributed through England and Wales, some 10 of them being "regional laboratories" in university centres, together with a central laboratory in London housing most of the reference laboratories. Before long the target number of laboratories was reduced to 60, but by 1950 the Chief Medical Officer was able to report that the PHLS was about three-quarters developed. This must reflect the energy and persistence (coupled it is said with some sleight of hand) with which Wilson set about persuading local authorities and hospitals to join in. Undoubtedly the offer of free public health microbiology services was a key factor in convincing local authorities that there was no need for them to finance alternative laboratories, and this aspect of the free service has never given rise to problems.

The decision that PHLS laboratories ought to be established in hospital premises called for negotiation not only with the hospital authorities but also with the consultant pathologists. In some cases new laboratories were established in hospital grounds without their being committed to provide bacteriological services for the hospital, but clearly there were great advantages if the PHLS laboratory in a hospital incorporated the hospital's bacteriological services, and this implied some sort of joint arrangement with the hospital. In his wish to get a comprehensive service developed as quickly as possible, Wilson often seems to have offered not only a free public health microbiology service but also a free, or nearly free, hospital microbiology service. For various reasons it was considered impracticable to ask hospitals to make a monetary payment for the services provided, so a variety of complex arrangements were made by which the hospital authority employed some of the staff – generally junior technicians – or contributed "in kind" in some other way. Over the years the demands for microbiology from the hospitals grew enormously but these barter arrangements very commonly lacked any arrangements for adjustment according to workload. None of this was a problem at the time, but when budgetary control of the PHLS became more stringent, and when the Department of Health required the Service to exact appropriate contributions from the hospital authorities, the disadvantages of pseudo-barter over a money economy became quite apparent.

Even with these financial inducements, and with the accepted high standards of PHLS work, it was not always easy to persuade hospital authorities, or particularly the pathologists in charge of the clinical laboratories, that surrender of the microbiology services to an "outside" organization was desirable. Indeed even with those who accepted, there was not infrequently some continuing strain arising either from envy or more general worry that the hospital staff played no part in the selection of the individuals who were to be their professional colleagues and who, it was expected, would have their main loyalty to the PHLS rather than to the hospital. It was not until 1962 that PHLS consultants were selected by a committee that included representatives of the hospital and the health authority.

During the years 1946–56, despite the economic crises and periodic bans on new building, a total of 44 laboratories were incorporated in the PHLS; 16 of these were county or municipal public health laboratories and three were newly constituted as separate public health laboratories. Twenty-four laboratories were established in hospitals but only 13 were initially to be responsible for a total clinical bacteriology service to a general hospital; the Bath laboratory (Figure 8) is an example of one that was not. Seventeen of the 44 laboratories had previously been associated laboratories, and two had been London sector public health laboratories. A "routine" diagnostic laboratory was set up in the Central Public Health Laboratory at Colindale to provide

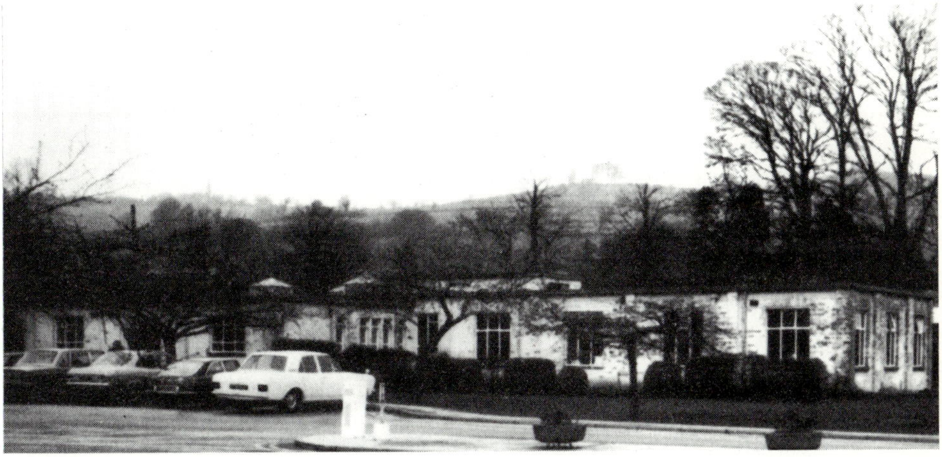

Figure 8 Bath Public Health Laboratory occupied part of this building from 1952.

a service to neighbouring boroughs similar to that offered by the area laboratories elsewhere. Many of the laboratories had to be established in premises that were far from ideal; several were improvisations in disused hospital wards. At Norwich one approach to the laboratory was through a cemetery – not conducive to work after dark – and at Epsom some of the rooms suffered from such extreme damp and dry rot that the director developed a fungal allergy.

The location of the laboratories was evidently determined by various factors. Obviously the aim was to provide laboratories so distributed that public health authorities throughout the county could have reasonable access to a PHLS laboratory. The opportunities and constraints that affected the achievement of this aim were certainly multifarious. Some local authorities had laboratories that were readily incorporated, but others cherished their own and did not wish to surrender them. Some hospital authorities invited Wilson to consider their site for a laboratory and some resisted the idea. In certain areas it must have been difficult just to identify a suitable location. The network, as it eventually developed, left few areas more than about 20 miles from a laboratory, but the populations in what might be regarded as the "catchment areas" of the various laboratories varied enormously: London and the Lancashire–Yorkshire conurbations have never had the number of laboratories that their populations might justify, and the southern counties have always been very generously provided. The war-time history provides a partial explanation; strong personal prejudices on the part of some pathologists in the North were certainly also an important determinant. It is perhaps curious that, when some contraction of the laboratory network was planned in the 1960s, four of the laboratories in the North were closed, so accentuating the north–south difference (see p. 125)

Laboratory building

Wilson's energies were not only directed to negotiating the incorporation of laboratories into the Service, or the establishment of new laboratories, but were also concerned with the design of the 22 new laboratory buildings that were put up between 1945 and 1961. To say that his concern was "intimate" would be a gross understatement; in fact he provided such detailed specifications and plans that he must be regarded as the *de facto* architect of many of the laboratories. In his "Historical notes . . ." there is a rather plaintive account of the difficulties encountered in the immediate post-war period. It had been agreed that all new laboratories should be built on hospital premises; the newly constituted hospital authorities were naturally concerned that any building for the PHLS should not obstruct the long-term development of the hospital, which had in any case often not been settled. Less reasonably, regional authorities sometimes insisted that their architects and engineers should be responsible for the design. In this, as in so many other fields, Wilson's persistence seems to have won through, and the laboratories he designed, though mostly now enlarged in various ways, form a fascinating series illustrating the development of his ideas, and of the needs of the laboratories (see Figure 9). He summarized these ideas in great detail in a paper

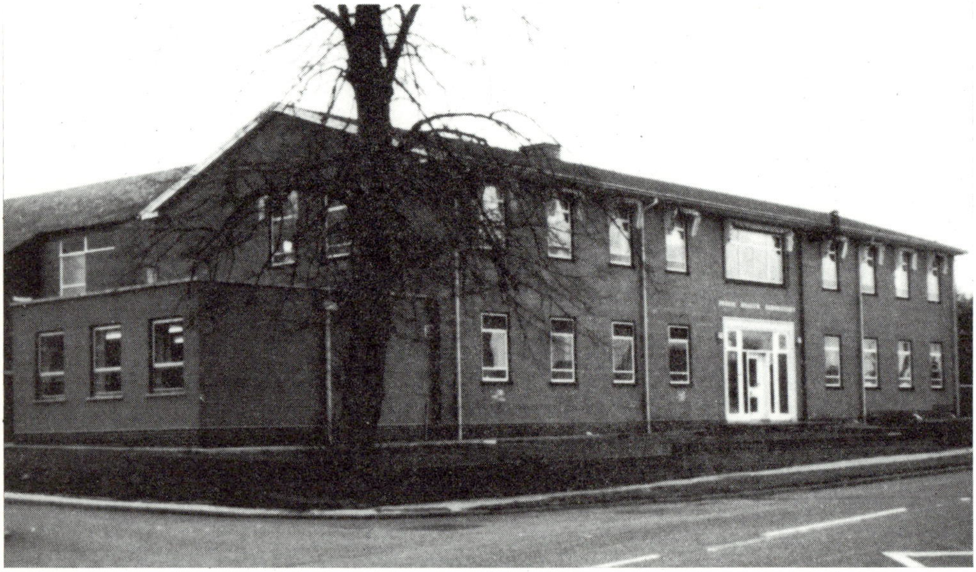

Figure 9 Chester Public Health Laboratory, opened in 1960, one of the last designed by Sir Graham Wilson.

privately printed at the London School of Hygiene and Tropical Medicine in 1967. His "signature", seen in many of the laboratories, comprised the use of a pinkish-brown brick, Granwood floors, ceiling lighting with the so-called "inverted brandy-glass" shade, and an entry corridor leading past offices and stores to a large laboratory, often with animal accommodation at the far end. The laboratory had window benches and a central service area. The generous animal accommodation dictated by the need to use guinea-pigs for the examination of milk for tubercle bacilli has provided a valuable area for expansion as the use of animals has declined.

Staffing

The staffing of an expanding service presented many difficulties. It was accepted that the directors of the constituent laboratories should all be medically qualified. In the early years individuals demobilized from the Armed Forces or returning to Britain from the Indian or colonial medical services constituted a valuable pool of recruits, but the universities were also expanding and attracting recruits from the PHLS and indeed the Annual Report for 1961 recorded the loss by then of seven staff to university chairs. Already in the war-time submission to the MRC, Wilson had detailed a scheme for training medical recruits; this was set into operation from 1946. It envisaged a five-year training period with about one year spent in a large hospital pathology or microbiology department and one year in an area PHLS laboratory, followed by an academic year attending the course for the Diploma in Bacteriology at the London School of Hygiene and Tropical Medicine (or later the similar course at Manchester) and then two years in either the Central Public Health Laboratory or one of the large regional laboratories. In essence this training scheme, which was a unique feature of the PHLS, survives to the present, being admirably suited to the preparation of trainees for the membership examination of the Royal College of Pathologists. Wilson encouraged trainees to develop some research project that would be suitable for an MD thesis, but a higher degree was not considered mandatory for promotion to senior positions.

Wilson selected all the trainees himself. Training posts were practically never advertised; individuals who wished to join the Service could apply to the Director, who would arrange to interview them. Many tales are told of these interviews. One successful applicant recalls it as being one of the most formidable experiences of his life, "with an interminable list of questions, far-ranging in the extreme". After an hour's interrogation, "almost totally lacking in humour", he was sent for an afternoon interview with Dr May Smith, a psychologist, whose kindly approach to a variety of aptitude tests was a welcome contrast to the rigour of the morning. Wilson was very anxious to get as full an understanding as possible of the personalities of potential recruits and to discover their motives in applying to join the Service. He has told me that Dr Smith's assessments virtually always confirmed his own. For those who were accepted as trainees, there was little option as to the laboratory to which they should be attached. Indeed appointment in the PHLS, even at a senior level, and even after the introduction of selection committees, included a condition to the effect that the "officer" could be moved from one laboratory to another at the discretion of the Director, or later the Board.

Trainees were interviewed by Wilson at various stages in their careers and although they were offered alternative laboratories for their next move, the choice seemed to many of them to have a strong "Hobsonian" element. But, although seemingly anxious not to reveal the fact, Wilson did actually try hard to reconcile the needs of the Service with the wishes or needs (perceived or not) of the individual. He was remarkably well informed on their personal situation as well as on their professional competence.

The "Dip.Bact." course at the London School of Hygiene and Tropical Medicine was, like the preliminary interview, intensive and exhausting, and it lasted for nine months, but the teaching was generally held to be very good and it undoubtedly gave the medical staff of the Service an academic background to their practical microbiology which was of immense value when they came to run laboratories on their own; it also gave them a substantial advantage over most of the hospital pathologists responsible for microbiology, for whom no comparable training was available. Wilson contributed to the teaching – he had of course been responsible with Topley for initiating the course before the war – and is recalled as lecturing, seated with arms crossed and eyes apparently shut, "selecting every word meticulously as though from a vast store-house in the depths of his mind, or as though reading from a manuscript in his mind's eye", and although he never used blackboard chalk, he always washed his hands before leaving the lecture room.

The laboratory staff were all employed by the Medical Research Council, except for a number of technicians employed by hospital management committees and allocated to PHLS laboratories under the cost-sharing arrangements already mentioned. After the Government had accepted the Spens report on medical salaries in the National Health Service, there were long discussions before it was finally agreed – in late 1949 – that the same salaries should apply in the PHLS. These differed from the university salary scales operated by the MRC for its research staff, a fact that later played a large part in convincing the Council that it should not continue indefinitely to administer the PHLS.

The MRC Board for the PHLS

The Medical Research Council had agreed to take on the administration of the PHLS for five years from the date of passage of the National Health Service Act of 1946; in 1950 it delegated administration of the Service to a Public Health Laboratory Service Board, with Dr A. Landsborough Thomson, then second secretary of the MRC, as its chairman (see Appendix Table 7).

Dr (later Sir) A. Landsborough Thomson (1890–1977, Figure 10) had been a member of the staff of the Medical Research Council since 1919 and as Principal Assistant Secretary was the administrator responsible to the Council for the running of the war-time EPHLS. His administration was in, or perhaps created, the liberal and non-bureaucratic tradition associated with the MRC at the time. He had been trained as a scientist, and was a superb administrator, whose first reaction to a request was not to consider possible objections, rather to enquire what he could do to help. He had the ability to see round or through problems, treating each on its merits, and achieve solutions, perhaps best summarized by his assertion that one should "play the rules according to the game". Landsborough Thomson established an immense rapport with Wilson and was perhaps Wilson's only confidant; together they effectively ran the PHLS until the establishment of the statutory Board in 1961, or indeed until both retired together in 1963. During this period the whole administration was on a purely personal basis; laboratory directors were able to approach the headquarters office directly and often solve problems or obtain urgent supplies with a speed that was the envy of those working in National Health Service laboratories, who had to work through committees and often experienced long delays.

The MRC Board was formally responsible to the Council for the activities of the

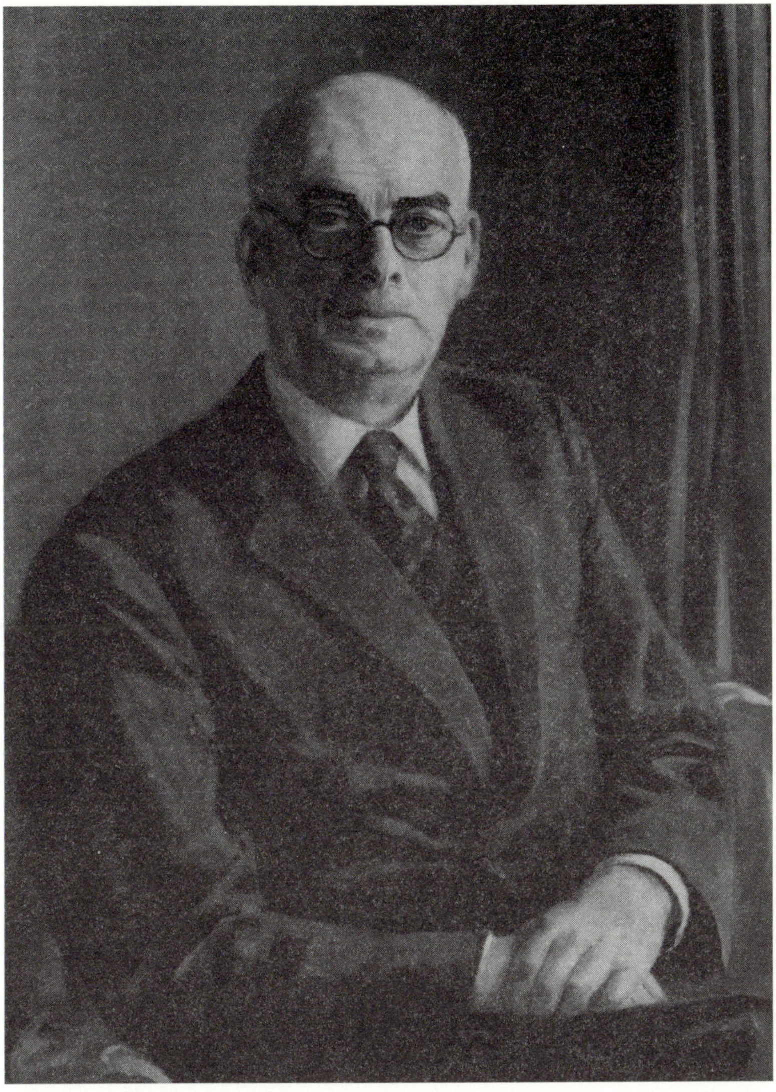

Figure 10 Sir A. Landsborough Thomson (from a painting by Peter Scott; reproduced with the permission of the Medical Research Council).

Service and for recommending appointments, but almost all its actions were determined by Landsborough Thomson and Wilson. Thomson once claimed that he not only chaired the meetings but also wrote the minutes, though it has to be said that that would not have been a difficult task as it consisted largely of putting the Agenda into the past tense: "The Board will be invited to consider . . ." became "The Board considered . . ." and little more. Although in the later discussions leading to the PHLS Bill it was stated that the policy of the Service was determined by the Board, practically the only policy discussions recorded in the minutes related to a redistribution of laboratories proposed in 1953 to accommodate the reduction in total number decided by the Ministry. And when the major changes in administration were being discussed during 1955 and 1956, the response was to cancel Board meetings "because of uncertainty on the future".

At first the Board had a small Appointments Committee to advise on consultant appointments, comprising Landsborough Thomson, A.A. Miles, H.J. Bensted, R.M. Fry and Wilson. In 1952 Bensted and Fry were appointed Assessors to the Board, and thereafter the Board itself made the appointments; as it only met once or twice a year these must have been largely retrospective.

The initial term of five years for which the MRC had agreed to administer the Service was due to terminate in November 1951; earlier that year the Ministry had convened a small committee to report on the current organization and activities of the Service. After three meetings this committee agreed a report in which the main conclusions included acceptance that a nationally organized bacteriological service was essential for the proper control and prevention of infectious diseases and that such a service was beyond the scope of local or hospital authorities. Two separate laboratory services were therefore necessary. At the same time, it was considered essential that there should be no overlap with services provided by local authorities or hospitals, and that where the volume of work was low one bacteriologist should suffice for both public health and hospital work (thus already blurring the concept of two services); where the workload was sufficient separate hospital and public health laboratories were justifiable. The general organization of the Service was considered appropriate, as was its involvement in applied research and in the field of sanitary bacteriology. The service should be provided free in respect of infectious disease, but charges might properly be made for work in connection with non-infectious diseases.

This reassuring report, received by the Chief Medical Officer of the Ministry in May 1951, justified the Ministry in asking the MRC to continue the administration of the Service for a further period. After discussion the Council agreed, in January 1952, to continue management of the Service for an indefinite period, terminable on six months' notice. The Council was warned that, in the light of the current financial stringency, development of the Service would be severely curtailed for the next few years, with a ban on new laboratory construction. The Ministry also asked that the conditions of service of the staff should be brought fully into line with those of the employees of the National Health Service – a request that caused considerable anguish when reported to the Staff Committee.

Relations with the Ministry of Health

The formative years of the 1940s preceded the era of multifarious advisory committees and of the burgeoning growth of the Ministry, and relations were at a senior and personal level. The Director of the PHLS attended the weekly policy meeting convened by Sir Wilson Jameson as Chief Medical Officer and continued in a slightly different form by his successors John Charles and George Godber, and the future organization of the PHLS was negotiated by Harold Himsworth (the Secretary of the MRC) and Landsborough Thomson, with the Chief Medical Officer and senior administrative officers of the Ministry. Wilson held regular meetings with the Ministry's consultant advisers, Panton and Bedson, on the relations between the PHLS and the hospital laboratory services, and he represented the PHLS on the Central Pathology Committee.

Charles Cockburn, who was in a better position than the rest of us to judge the situation, felt that the whole development of the PHLS owed a tremendous amount to the persistence with which Wilson's policy for the Service, and his relations with the Ministry, were governed by adherence to strict scientific principles and were not to be swayed by short-term political considerations; Cockburn doubted whether the Ministry always understood Wilson's ideas, but the very doggedness with which they were pursued triumphed in the end.

Relations with the Ministry and with the medical officers of health in connection with epidemiology were somewhat strained. Even during the war, Scott and Wilson had wanted to appoint epidemiologists but had been opposed by the medical officers of health and indeed by the Ministry, with the view that the laboratory service should confine itself to microbiology (although it was early agreed that the laboratories could engage in field work). After 1954 the Weekly Summary of laboratory reports contained material from the hospitals as well as from the PHLS and thus gave a very comprehensive account of the current prevalence of many infective diseases. Yet, when the medical officers of health asked to receive copies, the Ministry refused, partly on the grounds that the summaries contained some confidential information that might be withheld from a report having a wider circulation, but partly it seems reflecting the same feeling that the laboratory services should not reach out too far into the field of epidemiology.

Finance

This is a convenient point at which to interpolate a note on the cost of the PHLS. The details are given Appendix Table 6. From a figure of about £538,000 in 1948/9, the revenue expenditure rose to reach £1,165,000 by 1958/9. Capital expenditure fluctuated between £36,000 and £198,000, the larger sums being mostly for the new laboratory at Colindale.

The Staff Committee

A decision of the greatest importance in the establishment of the whole ethos of the PHLS was made as soon after the end of the war as October 1945: to establish a Staff Committee comprising the directors of all the constituent and reference laboratories. This continued a tradition of a number of informal meetings of senior staff held during the war, but the decision at the second meeting in December 1945 that the Committee should meet five times a year set a pattern that persisted almost unchanged until 1977, and even then changed only in detail. The meetings were at first held at the MRC office in Old Queen Street, Westminster, and from December 1945 to December 1952 at Church House, Westminster, after which they were held in the new library at the Central Public Health Laboratory, Colindale. The move to Colindale was not altogether popular with directors from outside London, if only because it meant that less time was available for other activities in the centre of the city. From the beginning, Staff Committee meetings were preceded by an informal buffet lunch and altogether contributed in a major way to establishing the *esprit de corps* that has characterized the PHLS for the last 40 years.

The meetings provided abundant demonstration of the varied characters whom Wilson had recruited to the Service. There were some directors who always sat in the front row, ready to intervene on most topics, some who, when the meetings were held in the Colindale library, found seclusion among the book stacks. There was Boycott (Figure 11) from Taunton, looking like a cross between a farmer and a bishop – justifiably in that he developed very valuable relations with the local veterinarians and also contributed to the satirical moralizing of *The Lancet's* Widdicombe File. In contrast, as an early member of the staff of one laborabory recalled, the day for a Staff

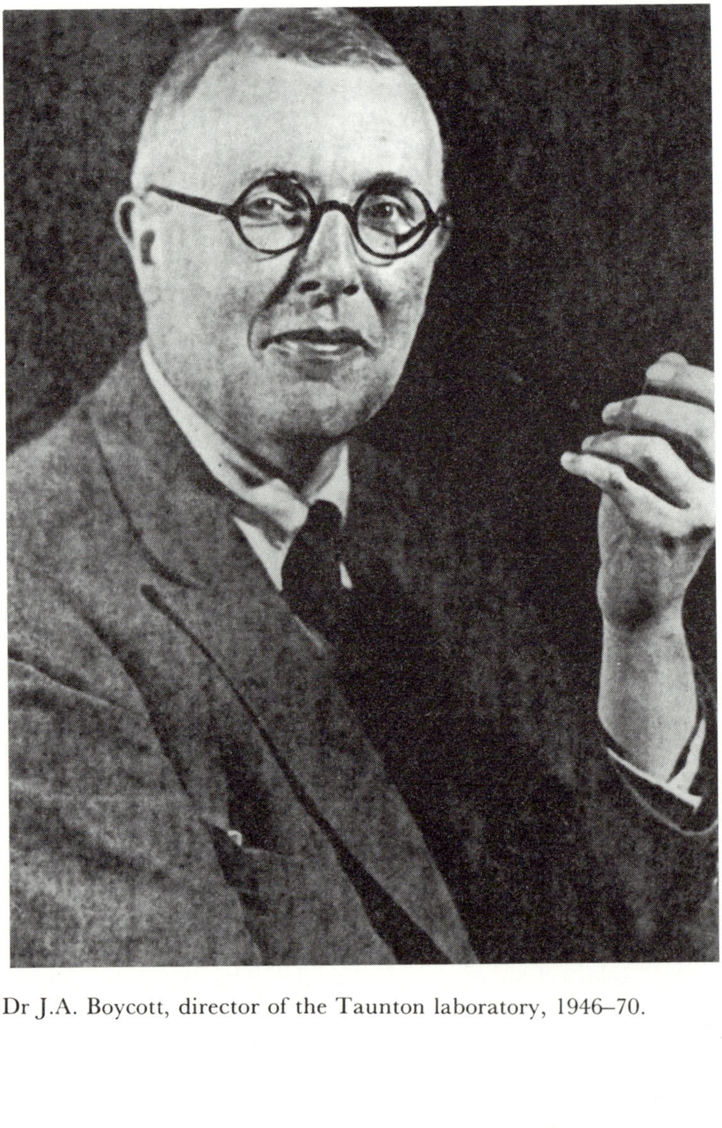

Figure 11 Dr J.A. Boycott, director of the Taunton laboratory, 1946–70.

Committee could always be recognized because his director appeared in a morning suit, Homburg hat and spats! It was indeed customary for lady members to wear hats. McCoy, from Hull, could always regale the Committee with the more sordid details of food production in agriculture. Tomlinson, from Bradford and later County Hall, London, was always ready to argue with authority, often (in the end) successfully. And, presiding over it all, Wilson, looking every inch the benign dictator (though sometimes, when arguments proceeded too long, with his eyes shut).

Early on the pattern was established that the meeting should commence with an extended discussion of some major microbiological or epidemiological topic. There would be time for discussion of smaller items of scientific or technical interest, followed by a period for administrative matters. Cynics claim that Wilson ensured that scientific discussions continued so long that enthusiasm was blunted when the time for administration was reached, and indeed members from more distant laboratories were leaving to catch trains.

The meetings of the Staff Committee were outstandingly successful in providing for the exchange of information and for enhancing the scientific and technical expertise of the laboratories. They gave opportunities for the release of steam by the directors present, and for the handing down of administrative decisions of the Director, or through him decisions of the MRC. Only to a very limited extent was the committee a decision-making body and, as seen from the floor of the meeting at least, it rather rarely appeared to influence administrative policy. On scientific policy it had more effect, particularly through the various technical subcommittees and working parties that it spawned (see Appendix Table 8), many of which published reports on methods or policies that were later recommended for use throughout the Service. But it was undoubtedly one of the strengths of the organization that the individual laboratory directors had a great deal of liberty to adopt the technical methods that they preferred, and the Staff Committee discussions enabled directors to review their own methods in the light of claims and problems advanced by their colleagues.

The Staff Committee meetings also gave directors an opportunity to call on members of the headquarters staff to press their needs, for more equipment or more staff – claims that were often settled one way or the other on the spot.

The Director's visits

Wilson reckoned to visit each laboratory in the Service at least once a year, and these visits gave further opportunities for discussion of technical methods as well as organization. The fact that all the staff in the laboratories saw the Director, even if distantly, on these occasions was also a valuable boost to morale. Wilson commonly arrived at the laboratory by bicycle, having taken the train only so far as would permit him to include a visit to some cathedral or church *en route*. This cycling sometimes presented problems, as when a laboratory director returning to his base to prepare for the visit, driving his rather old Rolls Royce, saw the Director of the Service pedalling along in front of him: to turn round, to pass at speed, or to offer a lift?

Wilson visited Colindale once a fortnight and called on all the reference laboratory directors; as he arrived in the late afternoon it was often late evening before he reached the last laboratory (which was generally Felix's Enteric Reference Laboratory) and there were very few other than the directors left to witness his visit.

Regional and area laboratories

The "master plan" envisaged about 10 "regional" laboratories situated in university centres. Although never set out very explicitly, it was thought that these laboratories would not only be larger, with more staff and resources and a wider range of services, than the "area" laboratories, but they would also be able to offer support to the area laboratories in their region, particularly with specialist tests and in providing locums from the pool of trainees that they expected to have. They might also be expected to organize local meetings and perhaps collate epidemiological intelligence. In actual fact, the regional laboratories, although commonly larger than almost all the area laboratories, have not developed the support roles envisaged; area laboratory directors have in particular cherished their direct access to the headquarters office and to the reference laboratories and epidemiological centre, and have not wished to see a tiered regional system. Association with universities has raised problems: university microbiology departments are already commonly accountable both to the university and to the hospital authority, and the addition of a third body is liable to cause, at least, confusion and, at worst, friction. In particular there is scope for dissension on the relation of the

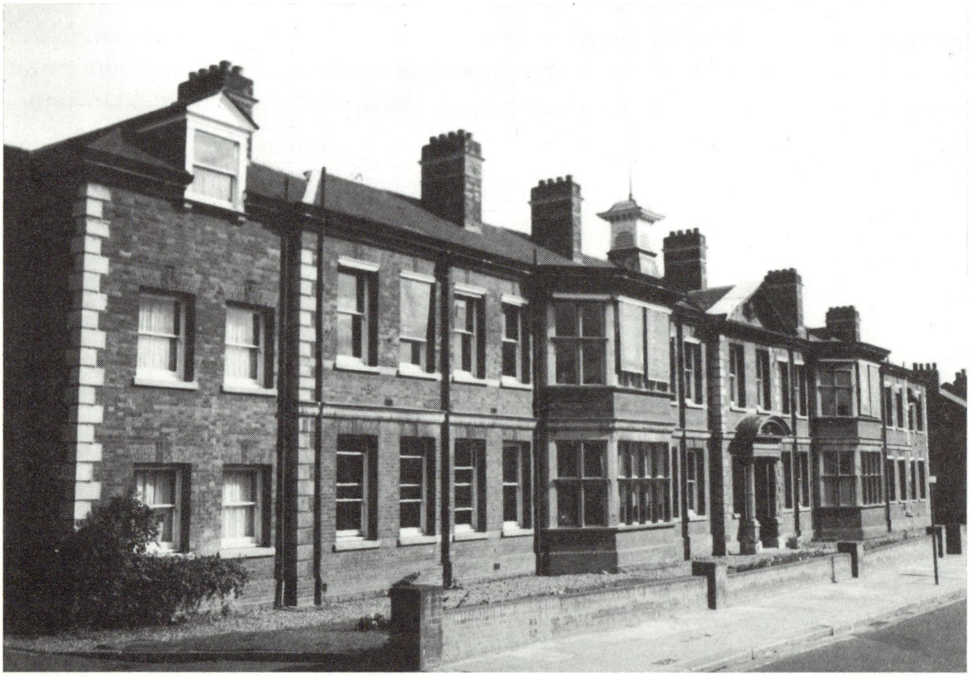

Figure 12 The Central Public Health Laboratory, Colindale: facade of the main laboratory block, *c.* 1980.

PHLS director to the professor, both posts normally free from any superior. The advantages that Wilson (1948*a*) saw for association of the PHLS laboratory with a university department probably work best if the association is at a reasonable arm's length.

In the text that follows I have generally used the term "area laboratory" to include area and regional laboratories.

Associated and recognized laboratories

To supplement the constituent laboratories of the PHLS a number of hospital and county laboratories were given the status of "associated laboratories" in the years up to 1946 (Appendix Table 3); the great majority were eventually absorbed into the PHLS. In the late 1940s, some 23 hospital laboratories were "recognized" (Appendix Table 4) and reimbursed from PHLS funds for any public health bacteriological work being carried out. Eleven of the "recognized laboratories" were within the area later covered by the Manchester, Chester and Preston laboratories; it was probably the strength of these local hospitals' interest in public health bacteriology that denied to the PHLS the opportunity of creating more constituent laboratories in the North-West. With the growth of the Service the number of "recognized laboratories" dwindled and there were none after 1972.

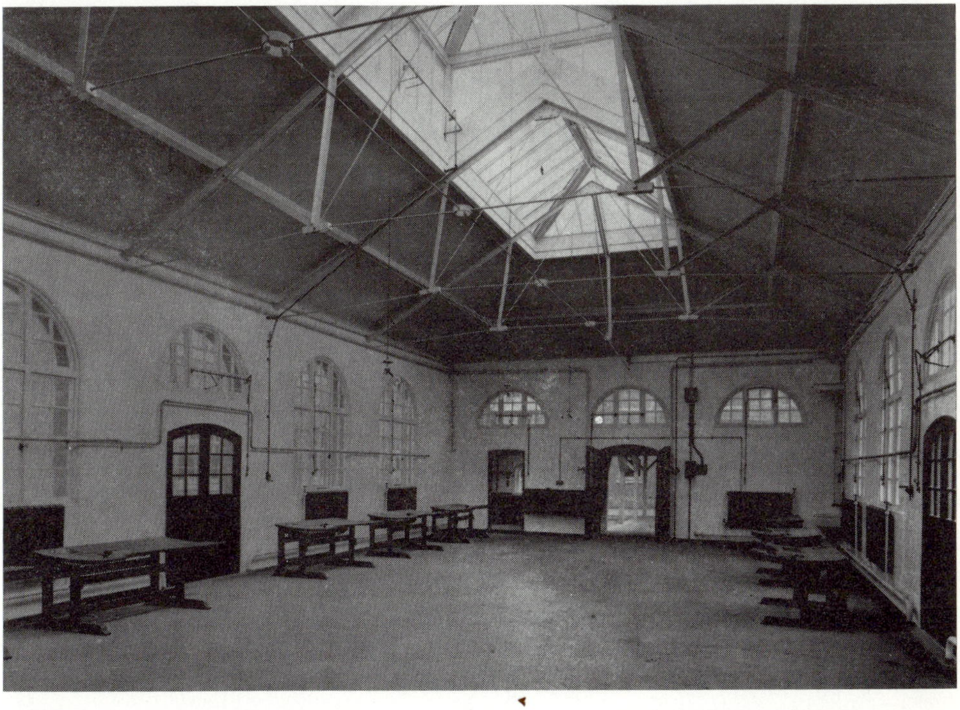

Figure 13 The operating hall of the Government Lymph Establishment, *c.* 1906: subsequently converted into the CPHL Library.

The Central Public Health Laboratory

A central laboratory comprising most of the specialist reference laboratories was part of the original plan for the post-war PHLS and it was fortunate that a substantial laboratory block became available at Colindale in North London at the end of the war. The Government Lymph Establishment, built with Edwardian solidity – and plumbing – in 1906 was handed over the PHLS in 1945, following the decision that smallpox vaccine production should be concentrated at the Lister Institute. The main laboratory block (Figure 12), on two floors, had 1442 m^2 of laboratory space and there were in addition on the 0.8 hectare site four substantial calf houses and a central block with 270 m^2 of floor area, which had been used for collecting the "lymph" from the skin of the inoculated calves (Figure 13). Dr Robert Cruickshank was appointed Director of the Central Public Health Laboratory (CPHL) and took up his post late in 1945.

Robert Cruickshank (1899–1974, Figure 14) had moved from Glasgow to London in

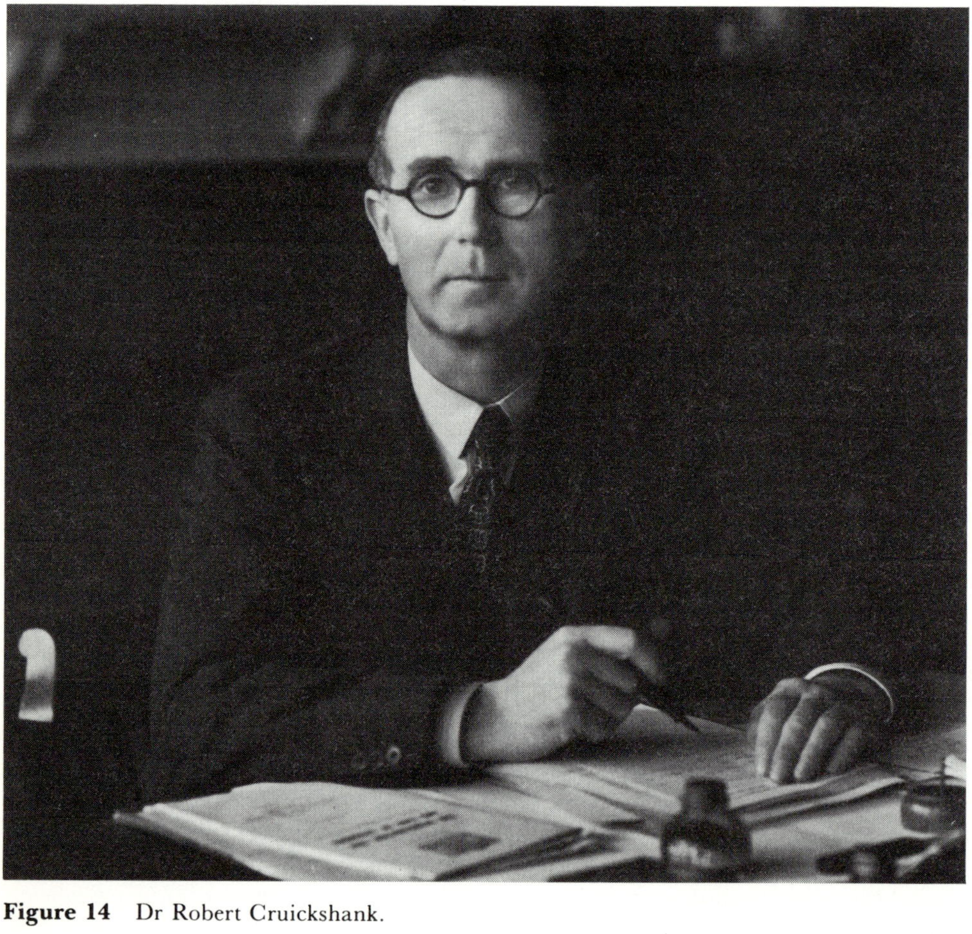

Figure 14 Dr Robert Cruickshank.

1936 to take charge of the London County Council Group Laboratory at the North Western Fever Hospital in Hampstead. This laboratory, as well as providing pathological services for a number of London County Council hospitals, was responsible for some public health bacteriology for neighbouring boroughs. Cruickshank was not only a very knowledgeable bacteriologist, but also had a great enthusiasm for epidemiological investigations coupled with laboratory work.

During 1946 the reference laboratories were assembled. The first was the Streptococcus Reference Laboratory, in January 1946. The streptococcal work, which had been Griffith's main interest in the Ministry laboratory before the Second World War, was largely concentrated during the war years at the Bernhard Baron Memorial Laboratories at Queen Charlotte's Maternity Hospital, London, where Leonard Colebrook had been studying streptococcal puerperal sepsis with the help of his sister Dora; Griffith returned from Cambridge to London in 1940 and directed the typing service until he was killed at the same time as Scott, in April 1941. S.D. Elliott, from the bacteriology department of the London Hospital, took over, but at the end of the war Elliott moved to New York to work with Rebecca Lancefield and decided to remain there for a time. The Streptococcus Reference Laboratory that opened at Colindale in 1946 was under the direction of V.D. Allison (see p. 12), who had worked with Griffith in the Ministry laboratory. He was supported by W.R. Maxted, as head technician; Maxted had worked with Griffith and with Elliott and was to be the sheet anchor of the laboratory for the next 35 years.

During the later war years Wilson, with J.D. Atkinson, who was appointed senior technical officer for the whole of CPHL in 1945, had developed the method for typing staphylococci with bacteriophages; Allison took this under his wing so that the laboratory became the Streptococcus and Staphylococcus Reference Laboratory. I joined the laboratory in 1946 and was soon involved in the trial of air-disinfection with ultra-violet that Cruickshank was planning (see p. 74).

The Virus Reference Laboratory was the second to arrive at Colindale, early in 1946. It was directed by F.O. MacCallum, a Canadian who had been a member of the staff of the Wellcome Research Laboratories and had played a leading part in the project for the production of a vaccine against scrub typhus during the war; he was also greatly interested in viral hepatitis and had done very valuable work on yellow fever. The first task of the Virus Reference Laboratory was to set up facilities for the laboratory diagnosis of smallpox (there were 56 cases in 1946), which had hitherto been available only in Professor Downie's department in Liverpool. MacCallum brought with him J.R. McDonald as head technician, and McDonald was to be a mainstay of the laboratory until 1981.

The Salmonella Reference Laboratory, under Joan Taylor (see Figure 26), had moved from Oxford to the National Institute for Medical Research for a short period at the end of the war; it too came to Colindale in 1946. Joan Taylor had been working at the Royal Free Hospital before the war and was one of the staff mobilized to the Oxford laboratory in September 1939. Her interests in serology fitted in well with Scott's work on salmonellas, so that she was soon helping him with the identification and took it over when he moved to London in 1940.

The Enteric Reference Laboratory had been constituted during the war for Felix to

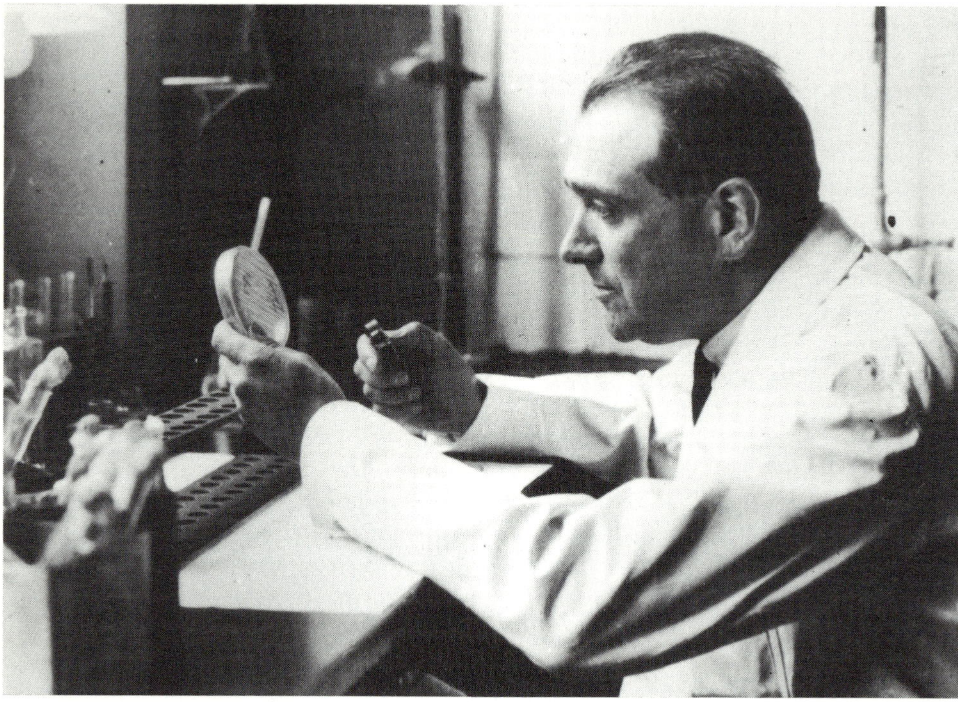

Figure 15 Dr Arthur Felix.

provide support for the investigation of typhoid and paratyphoid fevers (p. 21); it moved to Colindale in 1946.

Arthur Felix (1887–1956, Figure 15) had trained as a chemist; during the First World War he worked in the Austrian army on typhus fever and, with Weil, discovered the reaction now known by their names. After a period as a clinical pathologist in Palestine – he was a dedicated Zionist – he moved to the Lister Institute in London and worked on salmonella serology. He followed up some observations of Bensted's (p. 47) on the virulence and immunogenicity of typhoid bacilli for mice which led to the discovery of the Vi antigen and to the recognition that Vi antibody could be used as an indicator of the typhoid carrier state in man; this work was applied in Scott's investigations of the Croydon outbreak of typhoid fever in 1937. Felix's important work on phage typing has already been mentioned (p. 21) and the further exploration of the method, and its application to other salmonellas, was, with the setting up of the International Committee on Enteric Phage Typing, to occupy him for the next eight years. The International Committee was initiated at the Copenhagen International Microbiology Congress in 1947 and it was agreed that the Enteric Reference Laboratory should be the international reference centre, as it has remained. Felix was not an easy colleague; his obituary notice (Wilson, 1957) describes his mentality as "a curious cross between Central European and Oriental with the consequence that the workings of his mind were not always easy to follow". But what was easy to appreciate was the fact that once he had formed an opinion on some topic, he held on to it firmly and would admit no compromise; compromise he regarded as stupid. His "unshakeable confidence in his own judgement . . . occasionally led him into regrettable personal differences with other workers" – a statement that might have been put more forcibly elsewhere than in an obituary notice. This unshakeable confidence is nowhere better exemplified than in the fact that, to his death in 1956, he maintained that phages were enzymes produced by the host bacteria, not viruses. A more entertaining aspect of Felix's character was the obsession with which he carried bacteriological asepsis into his daily life: "Before he left the laboratory, he performed a lengthy ritual series of ablutions with hot water, soap and alcohol, which used to astound casual visitors, after which he could not bear to shake hands with anyone before taking food" (Wilson, 1957) and when on a visit to Israel with Wilson, advising on Israeli public health organization, he always wore grey cotton gloves when there was any likelihood of having to shake hands with anyone!

In 1947 Felix was joined by E.S. Anderson (Figure 22, p. 70) who had originally been appointed to work with Joan Taylor and who, so he told me, had early made a resolution never to work with typhoid; he had had considerable experience of outbreaks of enteric fevers in the Canal Zone during the war. Anderson soon revealed his abilities as an investigator by discovering "host modification" in the Vi phages used to type *Salmonella typhi*, although unfortunately Felix would not allow publication of the work and it did not appear until other workers had made similar observations five years later.

A laboratory for the production of standardized reagents for the laboratory diagnosis of typhoid and paratyphoid fevers had originally been set up at Oxford in 1915 and was subsequently financed by the MRC. Lt Col. R.F. Bridges was appointed to direct the Standards Laboratory, as it was now called, in 1939, and during the war years he collaborated closely with the Oxford EPHLS laboratory, in particular with Scott and Joan Taylor, in the preparation of diagnostic antisera for many salmonella serotypes. It was decided that this MRC Standards Laboratory should be transferred to the PHLS as the Standards Laboratory for Serological Reagents, and moved to the CPHL; it arrived during 1946 and Lt Col. H.J. Bensted was appointed its director.

H.J. Bensted (1888–1966) held a regular commission in the Royal Army Medical Corps from 1919 and, as well as periods at the Royal Army Medical College, he worked in Cairo and at the Enteric Laboratory at Kasauli in India. During the war he was Assistant Director of Pathology at the War Office. While at the College he had done pioneer work with the antigen thought to be essential for immunization against typhoid.

The work of the Standards Laboratory increased dramatically in the early post-war years, perhaps partly because it was decided that all material supplied to National Health Service hospitals should be free of charge (although the existing charge had not been changed since 1918!). It should be noted that the individual reference laboratories always prepared their own diagnostic reagents; those prepared by the Standards Laboratory were for issue to area and hospital laboratories.

The Food Hygiene Laboratory was opened early in 1947 with Dr Betty C. Hobbs in charge; she had worked with Wilson at the London School of Hygiene and Tropical Medicine and, during the war, with Allison at Cardiff. The idea for a food hygiene laboratory was probably largely Cruickshank's and from the first the emphasis of its work differed from that of the other CPHL laboratories in that it had a strong educational role. Cruickshank himself participated in several series of lectures, for which the Food Hygiene Laboratory prepared various exhibits, addressed to managers and staff of food-handling and catering establishments, and later public health inspectors. However, the laboratory also took on the routine "sanitary" bacteriology for the area covered by the Colindale Routine Diagnostic Laboratory (see p. 49) until that laboratory moved to the Central Middlesex Hospital in 1968, and it developed a number of reference services (e.g. serotyping of *Clostridium perfringens*) and research programmes.

The National Collection of Type Cultures, which originated as a reference collection of bacteria built up at the Lister Institute early in the century, was taken over by the Medical Research Council in 1920. It was transferred to the PHLS in 1946, although it was unable to move to the Colindale site until some new accommodation was available, in July 1949. The Collection was originally a repository of bacteria of many different sorts but in 1946 the decision had been taken that it should concentrate on bacteria of medical and veterinary interest. Dr S.T. Cowan (1905–76) was appointed Curator and initiated a systematic overhaul of the collection and transfer of the cultures from nutrient media to freeze-dried ampoules.

The remaining constituent unit of the CPHL in the late 1940s was the Epidemiological Research Laboratory. Dr W. Charles Cockburn was appointed to the PHLS in 1946 to organize and supervise the extensive field trials of whooping cough vaccine that were being planned by the MRC Whooping Cough Immunization Committee. It was not long before Cockburn became involved in a number of other epidemiological projects; he also took on the responsibility for editing the Weekly Summary of reports from laboratories.

From the early days of the war, a Weekly Summary had been prepared by Wilson from the weekly reports sent to headquarters from the EPHLS laboratories and was circulated to the laboratories, to the Ministry and to the Armed Services. Even after the work of compilation was taken over by Cockburn, the final report was always considered in detail by Wilson before issue. Cockburn recognized that the epidemiological value of the reporting system could be greatly enhanced if reports from National Health Service hospitals could also be included and so, during 1951, hospital pathologists were invited to contribute results from their bacteriological laboratories to the summary. The invitation involved Cockburn in the formidable task of identifying the appropriate pathologists and addressing some 400 individual letters, each of which was signed by Wilson. The response was encouraging, and with this development the Weekly Summary really started on its course towards becoming a major resource for the epidemiological study of infective disease in the country as a whole. Curiously, however, there was antagonism in the Ministry to making the information more widely available. It was not until many years later that the Weekly Summary's successor, the *Communicable Disease Report*, was sent to all the groups that had by then become known as medical officers for environmental health and chief environmental health officers.

There was, in the late 1940s, a degree of suspicion on the part of the medical officers of health that the growing epidemiological activities of the PHLS were encroaching on their territory; one is said to have remarked that "the cobbler should stick to his last and the bacteriologist to his bench". There was a similar fear in the Ministry of Health in respect of the epidemiological responsibilities of its medical officers. For these reasons, Wilson devised the title "Epidemiological Research Laboratory" for a unit that was no more, and no less, a research unit than any of the other reference laboratories. For the same reason, Wilson was unable to proceed with the plan for appointing regional epidemiologists. Nevertheless, it should be added that, over the years, both Cockburn in the Epidemiological Research Laboratory, and Wilson himself, were able to demonstrate the considerable help that an epidemiologically oriented laboratory service could bring to the medical officer of health, and they became accepted as colleagues, so that many valuable joint investigations were set up. Wilson was, indeed, later invited to join the Council of the Society of Medical Officers of Health.

Although the Central Public Health Laboratory was to be primarily a reference and research laboratory, a Routine Diagnostic Laboratory was established within the complex to provide public health bacteriological services for the surrounding boroughs and clinical bacteriological services for the Hendon Isolation Hospital. Its public health catchment area grew to include most of the London boroughs north of the Thames as well as a great part of Middlesex – a population of more than 3 million – and it came to provide a valuable resource for investigations sponsored by the Epidemiological Research Laboratory. The laboratory was, formally, directed by Cruickshank, but he was assisted by H.D. Holt, who was appointed director in 1947. There were also three "sub-laboratories", in Neasden and Coppett's Wood Isolation Hospitals and in the borough of Edmonton, where the PHLS took over a small "single technician" laboratory set up by the local medical officer of health. The Edmonton laboratory under Mair E.M. Thomas was particularly successful in attracting work from general practitioners. The medical microbiologists in charge of the three sub-laboratories each worked part of their time in the routine laboratory at Colindale.

At the third meeting of the Staff Committee, in February 1946, Cruickshank proposed the establishment of a Central Library for the Service, to be housed at Colindale but available for use by all laboratories. A system by which a selection of journals was circulated around area laboratories was developed and an allocation of funds provided so that each laboratory could set up a small library of its own. After one or two false starts, Miss Betty Whyte (Figure 16) was appointed Librarian and arrived early in 1948, to find a collection of some 800 volumes which Miss Wigmore (the MRC librarian) had acquired from the Metropolitan Life Assurance Sanatorium in New York, together with others discarded by the London School of Hygiene and Tropical Medicine and by the Harvard Hospital at Salisbury, as well as a few hundred left from the Government Lymph Establishment. This, together with subscriptions to some 85 journals, formed the nucleus of what has grown to become a quite outstandingly comprehensive library in the field of medical microbiology and epidemiology, having by 1977 some 20,000 journal volumes, 5500 books, and 450 serial publications a year. It was not until 1952 that anything like adequate accommodation was provided for the Library; in that year it moved into the central hall at the back of the laboratory building (illustrated before conversion in Figure 13). From 1949 a weekly bulletin listing relevant titles from journals received by the Library was circulated, at first within the

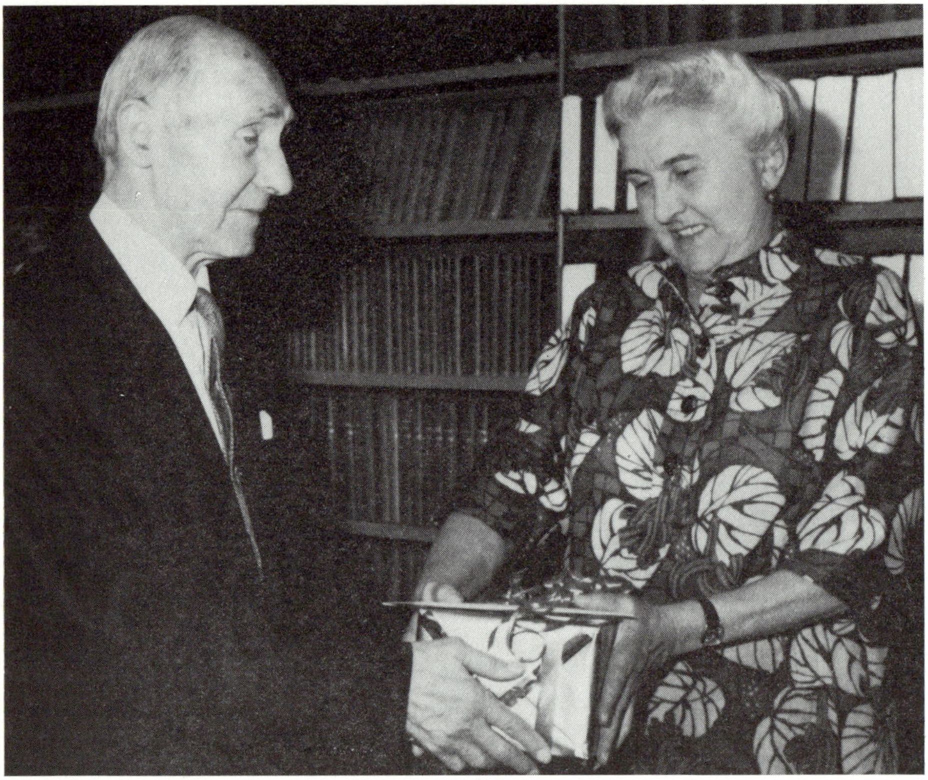

Figure 16 Miss Betty Whyte and Sir Graham Wilson at a party to mark her retirement in 1982.

Central Public Health Laboratory, then to all PHLS laboratories, and later to numerous other workers in Britain and overseas.

The position of the Director of the Central Public Health Laboratory was never very clear. Wilson's general philosophy was to leave to laboratory directors almost total responsibility for the scientific work of their units, and the reference laboratory directors were in any case senior individuals with long experience. Cruickshank already had a good many of those irons in the fire that were later to make him a peripatetic professor of bacteriology (and one who was in consequence able to give inestimable help in the field of communicable disease epidemiology in numerous countries throughout the world). As far as I am aware, Cruickshank made very little attempt to review or offer guidance or suggestions on the work of the individual reference laboratories, though he promoted very strongly some particular projects, such as the Food Hygiene Laboratory, the whooping cough vaccine trials, and the study of ultra-violet as an air disinfectant. Bensted, who succeeded Cruickshank in 1949, made even fewer excursions into laboratories other than his own; the periodic meetings of laboratory directors that he instituted were largely concerned with administrative matters. The facts that the Director of the CPHL did not have clear budgetary authority over the separate reference laboratories and that Wilson, at his fortnightly visits to laboratory directors, was prepared to consider directly requests for additional staff, certainly diminished the authority of the Director of the CPHL and there does not ever seem to have been any systematic reviewing of the total programme of the CPHL. The five Staff Committee meetings each year gave opportunities for the regional and area laboratory directors to make known their needs and any criticism of the reference services, but it was left entirely to the directors of individual reference laboratories to decide whether to heed these signals from the periphery.

Development of the Central Public Health Laboratory, 1946–56

The main developments in the CPHL in the first decade are summarized in Appendix Table 5. It was very soon evident that the laboratory space was inadequate, and also that the railwaymen's canteen at the nearby Colindale Underground Station needed to be at least supplemented by a café on the site. Two semi-prefabricated huts were put up in the garden, one of which was a canteen which may have been hygienic but certainly lacked elegance; the other was to house the National Collection of Type Cultures. Plans were also drawn up for a major extension to occupy an area of the garden that had, thanks to long cultivation supplemented by much calf manure, become a superb vegetable plot (Figure 17). Building commenced in 1951 and the laboratory was formally opened by Iain Macleod, the Minister of Health, in January 1953 (Figure 18).

At the beginning of 1949 Robert Cruickshank left Colindale to take up the chair of bacteriology, vacated by Sir Alexander Fleming, at St Mary's Hospital Medical School, London. He was actuated partly, we believed, by the Scotsman's innate respect for professorial chairs, partly by the fact that he would be following Almroth Wright and Fleming, and partly by the frustrations that he had experienced at Colindale, not

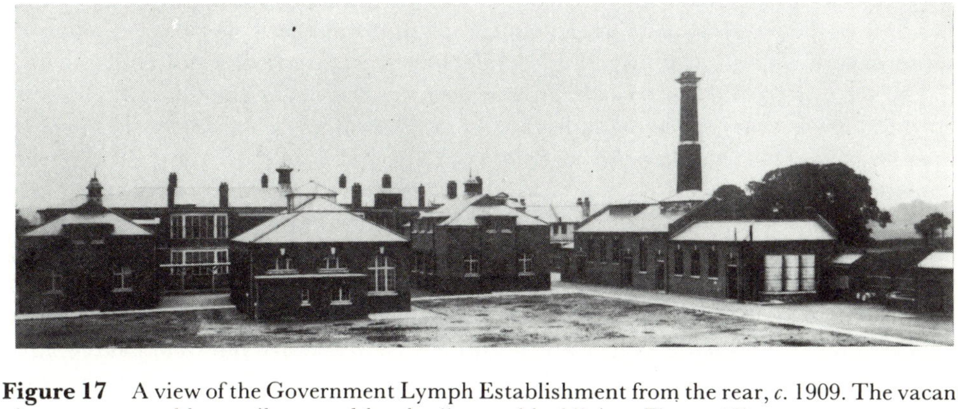

Figure 17 A view of the Government Lymph Establishment from the rear, *c.* 1909. The vacant plot grew vegetables until covered by the "tower block" (see Figure 18).

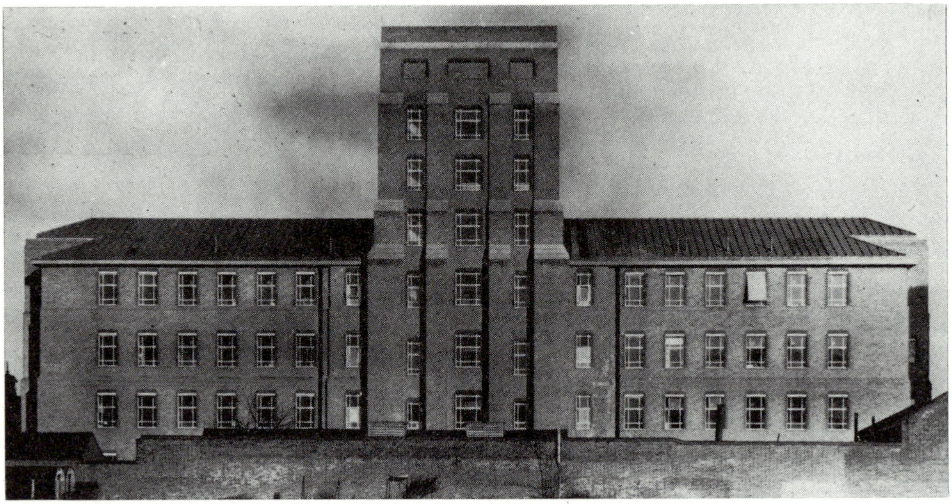

Figure 18 The "tower block" at the Central Public Health Laboratory, Colindale, 1952.

least in his dealings with Felix. Lt Col. H.J. Bensted, the director of the Standards Laboratory, was appointed to succeed Cruickshank, while retaining charge of his own laboratory.

V.D. Allison also left Colindale at the end of 1948 to take up a post of Senior Pathologist in Northern Ireland; I succeeded him as director of the Streptococcus and Staphylococcus Reference Laboratory. In 1952 we were joined by O.M. Lidwell, with whom we had already been working in the trial of ultra-violet air disinfection; Lidwell remained a member of the staff of the MRC, but a PHLS Air Hygiene Unit was constituted within the Streptococcus and Staphylococcus Reference Laboratory. Lidwell, whose original discipline was physical chemistry, had worked during the war years with R.B. Bourdillon and J.E. Lovelock; he brought to the laboratory a flair for devising and even constructing instruments that worked, coupled with a real understanding of the physical phenomena concerned in the airborne dispersal of microbes, and a deep if somewhat idiosyncratic understanding of statistics and epidemiology.

The serotyping of dysentery bacilli had been carried out in the Oxford laboratory during the war years, principally by Lt Col. R.F. Bridges, who was in charge of the Standards Laboratory; when the latter moved to Colindale in 1946, the dysentery work remained with Bridges in Oxford as the Dysentery Reference Laboratory. This laboratory moved to Colindale in 1952, when the new block was opened, under the day-to-day charge of Dr M. Patricia Carpenter, with, until 1956, Col. Bensted having overall responsibility for the laboratory.

In 1953 the Medical Research Council put up a large prefabricated barn adjacent to the Colindale site to serve as its Central Store with Mr Alan Waltho in charge; to an increasing extent this became the PHLS Central Store, and it was eventually transferred to the PHLS in 1977.

Reference laboratories outside Colindale

The Ministry of Health had, since the 1920s, supported a reference laboratory for venereal disease serology and around 1944 the unit was transferred to the PHLS as the Venereal Diseases Reference Laboratory. Dr I.N. Orpwood Price was appointed Director in 1945. The laboratory moved from the London School of Hygiene and Tropical Medicine, first to St Peter's Hospital, London E1, where it was housed in the mortuary block and a lecture room, the rest of the hospital having been destroyed by air-raids. There was no heating and a leaking roof. The laboratory hit the headlines when two rabbits infected with syphilis were stolen. After a period at the Eastern Hospital, Homerton, the laboratory moved to the new research block at the London Hospital in 1955. It was principally concerned with providing assistance and support for clinical laboratories performing serological tests for syphilis, and with testing (and in the earlier days preparing) the requisite antigens. It also acquired a very heavy first-line diagnostic role for the London Hospital's own VD clinic.

The Mycological Reference Laboratory was established at the London School of Hygiene in 1945, with J.T. Duncan as the first director; he was succeeded by R.W. Riddell in 1949. The laboratory developed very close relations with the Institute of Dermatology, and provided support for PHLS and hospital laboratories throughout the country.

The Malaria Reference Laboratory had been established by the Ministry of Health some years before the war to provide the infected mosquitoes used for the therapeutic induction of malaria in patients suffering from neurosyphilis; it was situated at Horton Hospital in Surrey and was transferred to the PHLS in 1948, with Sir Gordon Covell as director; he was succeeded in 1950 by P.G. Shute.

Another unit to be mentioned here is the Epidemiological Research Unit at Cirencester. Dr R.E. Hope Simpson, a general practitioner in the town, received financial support from the MRC for epidemiological studies in his practice population from 1947 and his "unit" is recorded as a "constituent laboratory" of the PHLS in the MRC Report for 1948–50, although the association with the rest of the PHLS was somewhat tenuous until the establishment in Cirencester of a small virological laboratory in 1960.

The Work of the Service, 1946–56

The scope of PHLS work

The PHLS entered the post-war era on the basis that it was set up to provide a free service covering any bacteriological laboratory work and related field investigations required for the diagnosis, prevention, and control of infectious diseases. "Infectious diseases" were thought of as those coming within the province of the medical officers of health, and the Service was essentially there to provide the laboratory support for the medical officers of health and their staff, particularly sanitary inspectors. The only regular supply of specimens from hospital in-patients would be from those in infectious diseases hospitals, and perhaps some maternity units separated from general hospitals, although it was envisaged that directors of the public health laboratories might have to take responsibility for organizing the examination of specimens of epidemiological importance for hospital laboratories in their areas. For reasons already mentioned (p. 29), it was also expected that diagnostic work related to venereal diseases and tuberculosis on patients in institutions would fall to the hospital laboratory service.

There was a running discussion on the distribution of tests for the purity of milk between the PHLS and the laboratories of the Ministry of Agriculture, Fisheries and Food, and there was limited discussion on the relations with the public analysts on tests for the purity of water, but the general principle was accepted that PHLS laboratories (and "associated" or "recognized" laboratories where appropriate) should test consumer specimens, while other arrangements had to be made for tests used to control production of safe water, milk or other food.

In January 1949 Wilson reported to the Medical Research Council on the development of the Service. By then most local authorities had begun to use the free PHLS service, although a few still maintained their own laboratories. The main problems facing the Service were recruitment of experienced pathologists, in the face of increasing competition from the hospital service, and difficulties in erecting or converting buildings for laboratory use. Nevertheless, the Service had attained some 70 per cent of its projected coverage, and was costing some £450,000 a year – a figure already higher than the original estimate for the costs of the complete Service (p. 26).

At the end of 1951 the Staff Committee was told of an "agreement" which Wilson had made with the Society of Medical Officers of Health, with the Ministry's approval, that defined the relation of the laboratory directors to the medical officers of health. This agreement stressed the statutory responsibility of the medical officers of health for the control of infectious disease and the need for the laboratories to act only in support of, or at least with the concurrence of, a medical officer of health; the PHLS was not to initiate any field investigation (other than with general practitioners) without the prior agreement of the local medical officer of health. Wilson added that he had emphasized to the Society that the field epidemiologists whom he hoped to appoint to the PHLS would amount only to a few special officers for research purposes (cf. p. 49). The Staff Committee was concerned that too many concessions had been made to the susceptibilities of the medical officers of health who, it was recognized, had suffered by the loss of some of their clinical responsibilities in the terms of the National Health Service Act. The directors also suspected that the Ministry might be somewhat equivocal in its support of the PHLS.

The principles governing the work of the PHLS were set out by Wilson in his Milroy Lectures delivered to the Royal College of Physicians in 1948 (Wilson, 1948*a*). He quoted Dr Milroy's will as a reasonable text for the PHLS: "to determine the part played by contagion in the development and spread of various diseases [which] can only be effected by the patient investigation of numerous *verified* and *authenticated* facts in various localities and regions, and under different circumstances and conditions . . .". Wilson concluded that the two subjects of hospital pathology (including bacteriology) and public health bacteriology were essentially distinct, that they had grown up with different historical backgrounds and that their association in a single laboratory was fraught on the whole with deleterious consequences for preventive medicine. He saw hospital bacteriology and public health bacteriology as separate branches of pathology under different technical control, one caring for the individual, one for the herd.

Most of the PHLS laboratories operating in 1948 were indeed distinct from the hospital clinical pathology laboratories, which at that time were mostly directed by pathologists practising more than one discipline of pathology. But a major theme in the evolution of the PHLS has been the gradual blurring of the distinction and it is interesting that Dyke, in a perceptive note published in 1941, which he subsequently related (see Foster, 1961) had been written after discussion with Topley, pointed out the fallacies implicit in too rigid a distinction of hospital and public health bacteriology: one specimen could be equally important for the clinical management of the individual and for the epidemiological management of the community. The fact that it had been decided that the public health laboratories should, as a general principle, be established on hospital premises inevitably had the consequence of calling in question the distinction between clinical and public health bacteriology.

The relations between the public health laboratories and the hospital laboratories were a continuing topic of discussion for several years. On the one hand the PHLS directors were concerned that, with the absorption of the infectious diseases hospitals and independent maternity units into general hospitals, clinical microbiological work would be lost to the PHLS. On the other hand, hospital pathologists were concerned by what they saw as encroachments by the PHLS into their territory. A meeting was convened at the Ministry in August 1947, with the Chief Medical Officer in the chair and with representatives of the PHLS and of the hospital pathologists present. Dyke, a leading clinical pathologist, regarded the separation of the PHLS from the hospital laboratory services as dangerous and liable to lead to confusion; there were too few pathologists to man separate services, and to have the two services working side by side in a single pathology "centre" would lead to difficulties in administration and discipline. The PHLS representatives maintained that public health bacteriology was a separate branch of bacteriology and demanded men with qualifications and skills beyond those of the hospital bacteriologist. The Chief Medical Officer made the point that the PHLS had been established to meet the inadequacies of the existing situation, in which there had been no organization able to undertake field work or to provide early information for the medical officers of health. The report of the meeting concludes that there was a "degree of general agreement", and a memorandum was eventually issued in July 1949 indicating that all examinations related to outbreaks or suspected outbreaks of infection should be referred to the PHLS and not to hospital laboratories, and that all "sanitary" bacteriology should be done by the PHLS. It was later confirmed that work for infectious diseases hospitals should also be sent to the PHLS. The somewhat peremptory tone of the intimation that hospital laboratories should "inform the public health laboratory" of outbreaks, and send a weekly report of numbers of cases of certain specified infections, is a reflection of the insecurity that the PHLS was experiencing, and of its confidence that it could pursue outbreaks of infection much more effectively than any hospital laboratory. It was finally accepted that, though the PHLS should not undertake hospital bacteriology unless specifically asked to do so, heads of laboratories should be prepared to act in a general supervisory or consultant capacity in nearby hospitals. The implication of the superior quality of the bacteriological work in PHLS laboratories in this decision certainly reflected the belief of many members of the Service and was probably, at that time, justified. Directors were also encouraged to seek appointment to local pathology advisory committees. Wilson himself represented the PHLS on the Ministry's Central Pathology Committee.

A paper in the MRC files summarizes the views of several PHLS laboratory directors on the relation of the clinical and public health laboratory work, and the unsigned and rather confused summary suggests that the view that the two cannot be artificially divided was probably nearest to the consensus; although the sanitary side was linked with the medical officer of health and the clinical side with the hospital, a large part of bacteriology was common to both. However, bacteriology was inseparable from prevention and when considered as a whole was held to be no more a part of clinical pathology than social medicine, industrial medicine or epidemiology. The dilemma was best solved, it was suggested, by putting hospital bacteriology under the technical direction of the public health bacteriologists, although there should be two laboratories – clinical and public health – in one building, each with a director having full freedom to run his laboratory! It is no wonder that the next two decades were to see great variety in the pattern of relations between the public health laboratories and the hospital service.

At this time the work of the average public health laboratory consisted very largely of the examination of specimens from medical officers of health, sanitary inspectors and general practitioners. General practitioners had been encouraged to use the free services provided by the PHLS for tests on patients suspected of infectious diseases from early in the war years and this "open access" long antedated similar facilities in the hospital laboratories. Although the proportion of practitioners who used the service was generally small, some were very keen and productive associations developed that formed the nucleus from which several group research projects grew. Both general practitioners and sanitary inspectors were regular visitors to the laboratories and the directors were in regular communication with the medical officers of health. Field investigations in schools, day nurseries and among the general public (in the case, particularly, of outbreaks of food poisoning) were commonly undertaken.

By 1952 there was concern that the demands on PHLS laboratories for antibiotic susceptibility tests, particularly on tubercle bacilli, were growing. Wilson had agreed with Bedson, the Ministry's consultant adviser, that susceptibility tests ought to be the responsibility of the hospital laboratories: "their numbers should not be allowed to interfere with the legitimate work of the laboratories"!

The relations with hospitals and with the medical officers of health came up yet again in 1953. It was a long-standing tradition in the PHLS that when a laboratory recognized a pathogen in a specimen it reported the fact to the medical officer of health, even if the specimen had been sent from a patient under the care of a general practitioner. A problem arose when the patient was in a hospital, and the hospital did not wish the medical officer of health to be informed – an illustration of the reluctance of hospital staff to accept help from the medical officer of health in controlling infection.

In February 1955 the Staff Committee returned to the topic of "the work of the Service", with a paper by Tomlinson on the problems of research; the capacity of the PHLS for research had, it will be recalled, been a prime argument in persuading the MRC to continue with its administration. Research could be "individual", "collaborative" or "directed", and it was thought that collaborative research was particularly appropriate for the PHLS, and was probably best organized through the Staff Committee. Indeed, over the years, the committee certainly stimulated and co-ordinated a great number of collaborative research projects, many of which will be mentioned later.

But the discussion widened from research to an expression of worry over the consequences for the PHLS of the development of the National Health Service. In connection with a concurrent discussion over salary scales, Wilson had said that the PHLS was not a part of the National Health Service – an assertion that caused considerable dismay, but nevertheless justified the continuation of some privileges denied to National Health Service staff. It was held that the development of the hospital services independently of the PHLS was tending to take work away from the PHLS laboratories; there seemed to be a risk that small laboratories might be left with no more than the sanitary bacteriology. The response to this concern, in 1955, was to stress the fact that the strength of the PHLS lay in the service, including research, that it could give to the medical officers of health, general practitioners, the MRC, and various Ministries, and that this should continue to be its main function. The opportunities open to the PHLS in diagnostic virology and epidemiology were also seen to be considerable. Moreover, as Wilson pointed out, despite the claim that work was being taken away, the actual number of specimens examined in the laboratories had increased.

Laboratory workload is notoriously difficult to measure and several attempts have been made, during the lives of the EPHLS and the PHLS, to devise acceptable methods for such measurement, without much success. In a paper prepared for the Ministry's

1951 review of the functions of the Service, the following figures are given for the numbers of specimens received:

for 1947, with 28 laboratories,	468,295;
for 1948, with 35 laboratories,	789,901;
for 1949, with 44 laboratories,	981,400;
for 1950, with 46 laboratories,	1,180,617.

In an average week, in 1950, "medical" specimens amounted to 12,000, "venereal disease" specimens to 4500, "sanitary" specimens to 4000, and "miscellaneous" specimens to 2500.

From 1955, figures are available for numbers of specimens received, categorized by the nature of the investigation to be undertaken. Some of these figures are abstracted in Table 2 and the whole series is illustrated in Figures 37–40 (pp. 167–170). It will be seen that, by 1957, the total number of specimens had risen to 1,786,000, about 20 per cent being "sanitary" specimens.

Table 2 Numbers of specimens received by PHLS laboratories, in thousands

Year	Total	Isolation from "human" sources		Serology	Sanitary
		Bacteria	Viruses		
1947	468	NA	NA	NA	NA
1950	1181	NA	NA	NA	*c.* 208
1957	1786	1111	29	286	361
1969	3518	2781	71	599	505
1980	5923	3931	166	1519	289

NA, not available.

In the rest of this chapter the work of the Service has been summarized in relation to the prevalent infections. The annual reports of the Chief Medical Officer for England and Wales have been taken as the text on which to develop an account of the ways in which the PHLS laboratories reacted to the infectious diseases, and the ways in which they contributed to their control.

Smallpox

For many years the first entry in the chapter on epidemiology in the annual report of the Chief Medical Officer of the Ministry of Health was concerned with smallpox, the last of the "quarantine diseases" to be endemic in Britain. The Virus Reference Laboratory had, as a major element in its initial remit, the establishment of a laboratory diagnostic service for smallpox, and an announcement of the availability of the service appeared in the *Monthly Bulletin of the PHLS* in January 1947. At the time reliance had to be placed on complement fixation tests on vesicle fluid as a rapid (18–24 hour) method to supplement culture in the chick embryo; the much more rapid agar-gel precipitin method was not used until 1959. In the smallpox epidemics of 1946 and 1947 several members of hospital medical and nursing staffs were infected; the epidemics mostly originated from missed cases, often individuals who had modified disease due to partial immunity. By 1948 Murray and Bradley, writing from the Ministry, were able to assert that positive laboratory reports ought to over-rule hesitant clinical opinion (see MacCallum, 1952). And in 1950 laboratory tests at Colindale and Liverpool provided great help, not only in identifying the first case in an epidemic in Brighton, but also in helping to show that a large group of suspects associated with an incoming ocean liner were suffering from chickenpox, not smallpox. The year 1952 saw an epidemic with 135 cases of variola minor in Lancashire; it was suspected that the virus might have been imported in bales of cotton. Cotton was also suspected as the vehicle in an outbreak of variola major in Lancashire in the following year, and MacCallum set up several laboratory studies of the survival of virus in crusts from smallpox patients mixed in with cotton (MacCallum and McDonald, 1957). Although importations of smallpox resulting in small numbers of cases occurred in several succeeding years, in only two years (1962 and 1966) were these of any large number.

From 1946 PHLS laboratories were responsible for holding stocks of vaccine lymph for issue to medical officers of health and practitioners.

Typhoid and paratyphoid fevers

Although the numbers of cases of typhoid and paratyphoid fevers had declined substantially by 1946, typhoid in particular was still a serious disease, with some 10 per cent mortality. The use of phage typing showed that the classical case of "Typhoid Mary" was by no means untypical and that the existence of long-term symptomless carriers could explain a number of what appeared to be unrelated sporadic cases. Phage typing was on occasion able to confound what appeared to be a clear epidemiological picture, as at Oswestry, where the strains from patients with typhoid proved to be of a different phage type from that of the putative source – a chronic carrier who could have contaminated raw milk. In fact the outbreak was shown, many years later, probably to have originated from imported canned meat (Anderson and Hobbs, 1973). But the recognition of the importance and prevalence of chronic carriers, and the occurrence of a large outbreak of typhoid at Aberystwyth in 1946 shown to originate from a chronic carrier, appears to have been the stimulus to set up an organization that Felix had proposed in a private note in 1944. The Enteric Reference Laboratory was given the task of compiling a register of all human chronic carriers of *Salmonella typhi* with the idea that this might provide a means of prevention ("eradication" in Felix's note); the laboratory henceforth included the word "Bureau" in its title.

The phage typing employed for epidemiological purposes also had a spin-off at the more fundamental level: the observation in the Kilcreggan outbreak of 1948 – attributed to a chronic carrier presumably infected in 1895 – of two different phage types of *S. typhi* led to Anderson's discovery of the "type-determining" phages and the demonstration that the phage type of a clone of *S. typhi* was not immutable.

The Enteric Reference Laboratory was active in standardizing methods of serological diagnosis, which formed the topic of Staff Committee discussions in 1948 and 1949,

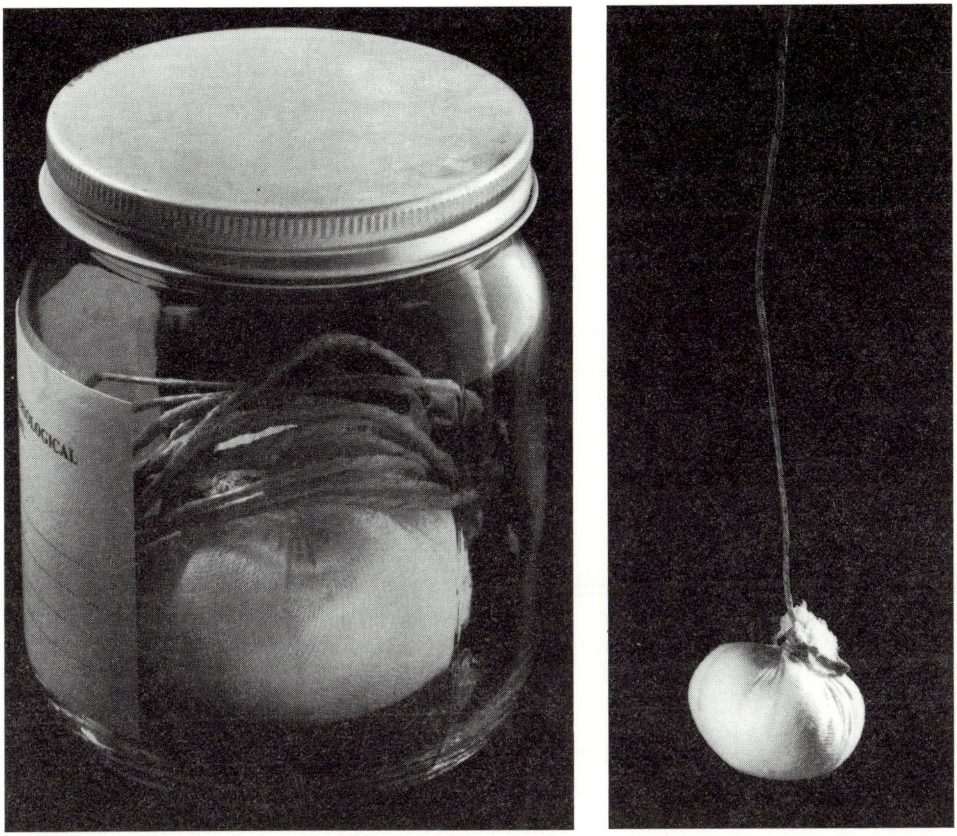

Figure 19 Sewer swabs used by Harvey in the Cardiff laboratory and developed from Brendan Moore's original design (cf. Figure 20).

and further developed the phage typing of *S. typhi, S. paratyphi* and *S. typhimurium.* Various laboratories participated in trials of chemotherapy both for the acute disease and for chronic carriers. Chloramphenicol was not available until 1948 (and at a Staff Committee in 1949 Felix is recorded as having deplored the number of papers extolling its virtues!). In the meanwhile several trials were made of penicillin and sulphathiazole, one benefiting from the large number of cases of typhoid occurring in the Aberystwyth epidemic (Bevan *et al.*, 1948). Moore (1948) described the use of cotton gauze swabs suspended in flowing sewage as a method of tracking carriers (Figure 19); by sampling sewers at different points it was possible on occasion to identify the actual house in which a carrier was residing (Figure 20).

When Anderson took over the direction of the Enteric Reference Laboratory and Bureau in 1954 he told Wilson that he intended to expand the laboratory's interest in the typing of *Salmonella typhimurium*, the commonest salmonella serotype, for which a scheme had been developed in the laboratory (later published by Callow, 1959), and to link the epidemiology of the infections in man with those in the animal population.

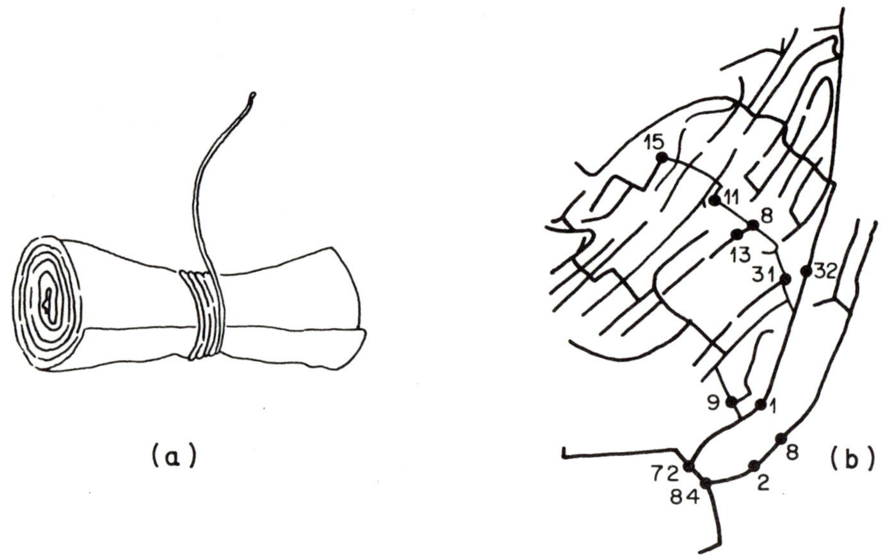

Figure 20 Use of a sewer swab to locate salmonella carriers: (a) diagram of the original type of sewer swab as developed by Brendan Moore; (b) sampling points used on a sewerage system – numbers refer to numbers of salmonellae isolated from swabs at each point on the system (redrawn after Harvey *et al.*, 1969). (See also Figure 19.)

Although Wilson was chary of this expansion, he allowed it to proceed – fortunately, because the link led to many advances in epidemiology and molecular biology (see p. 147).

Bacterial food poisoning

Bacterial food poisoning has inevitably been a major preoccupation of the Service from the start, but the first post-war decade witnessed an astonishing increase in the number of incidents reported to the PHLS, from 675 in 1946 to 4547 in 1956. It is difficult to know how much of this increase represents a real change in the incidence of illness. These figures refer to incidents (sporadic cases or outbreaks) in which material was sent for examination in a laboratory and gave evidence that the patient's illness was due to one of the recognized bacterial causes of food poisoning. Incidents with no bacterial, or viral, cause ascertained amounted to some 3000 in 1956 but systematic study of these incidents had to wait until the late 1970s. The increase in laboratory facilities, and the enthusiasm of laboratory directors, must be in part responsible for the increased number of reported incidents. But, in the words used in the Chief Medical Officer's report for 1955, we were in the midst of a catering revolution with a great switch from individual to communal catering, a switch calculated to foster the conditions that can lead to food poisoning, but one also conducive to the reporting of the incidents that occur.

Around 1947 Cockburn initiated a system for the central collection and analysis of the information on food-poisoning incidents received from the area laboratories and its collation with information on the incidents emanating from the Salmonella, Staphylococcus and Enteric Reference Laboratories and the Food Hygiene Laboratory. The "Annual reports on food poisoning in England and Wales", prepared for 25 years by Mrs Enid Vernon (later Hepner) give a superb view of the changing pattern of disease over the years (see, for example, McCoy, 1975; see also Figure 21).

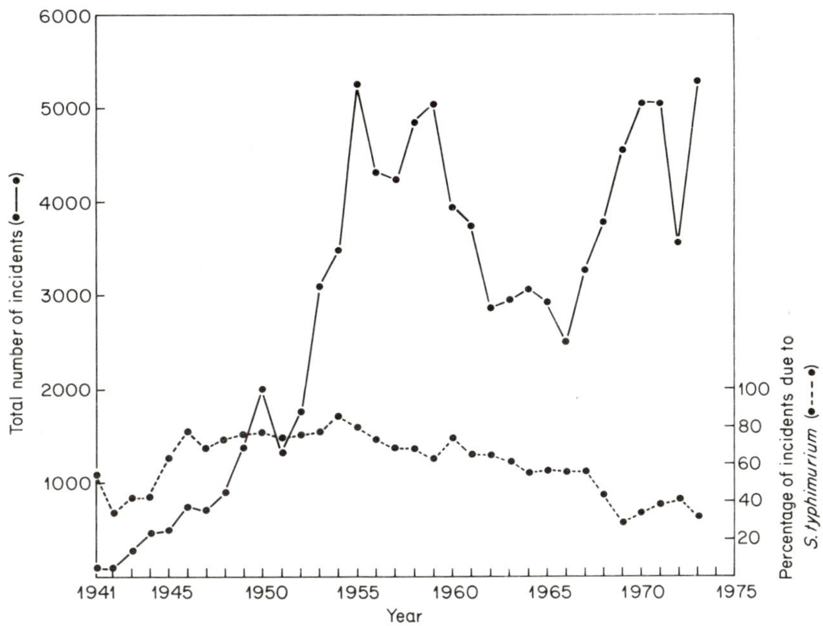

Figure 21 Numbers of incidents of salmonella food poisoning reported to the EPHLS and the PHLS, 1941–72 (after McCoy, 1975).

Infections due to salmonellas, especially *S. typhimurium*, were always the most numerous. The recognition of dried egg imported from the United States during the war as an important reservoir for salmonella food poisoning has already been mentioned as one of the achievements of the EPHLS. Even after American dried egg had ceased to be imported, egg-derived salmonella food poisoning remained in various forms. Outbreaks attributed to duck eggs feature in the records for 1947, 1948 (in a London hospital), 1951 and 1953; in 1953 a study found 15 per cent of duck eggs to harbour salmonellas.

In 1948 there was an explosive outbreak of paratyphoid fever in Eastbourne, due to a strain of *Salmonella paratyphi*, phage-type Taunton; the vehicle of infection was shown to be synthetic cream, although the source of contamination was not discovered (Cockburn, Jameson and Fenton, 1951). Subsequently synthetic cream was shown to be the vehicle in a good many outbreaks of paratyphoid fever and food poisoning. In 1955 the PHLS Salmonella Committee started an extensive examination of processed eggs and egg products, and found that many batches contained salmonellas; among the most heavily contaminated were frozen egg and albumen imported from China and in these *S. thompson* and *S. paratyphi* were frequently discovered (PHLS, 1958*a*). These egg products were widely used in bakeries and it was suggested that the salmonellas were transmitted to synthetic cream and other unheated foods by contamination of equipment and the environment. These observations offered an explanation for the hitherto mysteriously high prevalence of *S. thompson* food poisoning, for which there were no readily recognizable indigenous sources, and for many of the cases of paratyphoid fever. Indeed, of 20 phage types of *S. paratyphi* from cases investigated in 1955 and 1956, the eight found in Chinese egg had been responsible for 80 per cent of the incidents (PHLS, 1958*a*). These studies thus confounded the long-held idea that outbreaks of paratyphoid fever occur in the vicinity of the carrier who is the source; the bacilli can evidently travel far in space and time if they are introduced into egg products.

The Food Hygiene Laboratory and the Ministry of Agriculture, Fisheries and Food Laboratory at Cambridge developed heat-treatment methods for both albumen and liquid egg, and tests for the efficacy of the pasteurization. Regulations requiring heat treatment of egg products were introduced in 1964 and this particular source of food poisoning was eliminated; there were of course plenty of other sources already extant, or awaiting discovery or development (see p. 145).

The period also saw considerable interest in staphylococcal food poisoning and the recognition that, in contrast to salmonella infections, the staphylococci were almost always derived from a human carrier. This demonstration was greatly assisted by the development of phage typing for staphylococci and the setting up of typing services in a number of laboratories. Phage typing also showed that the staphylococci responsible for food poisoning generally belonged to one or other of a small number of phage types (Williams *et al.*, 1953). The vehicle of staphylococcal food poisoning, though sometimes a meat product, was often some "sweetmeat", cream cake or ice-cream. The importance of ice-cream, often manufactured on a small scale with quite inadequate hygiene, was recognized quite early and the PHLS set up a particularly active subcommittee, under E.H. Gillespie, on the bacteriological testing and grading of ice-cream. It issued four reports in as many years which provided guidance on hygienic methods for the production of ice-cream and showed that the methylene blue test could be used as an indicator of effective treatment. Eventually the Ministry of Health made regulations requiring heat treatment of the ingredients of ice-cream.

A series of outbreaks of toxin-type food poisoning attributable to spray-dried skim milk occurred in 1953 and involved nearly 1200 cases; examinations in several PHLS laboratories revealed a high level of contamination of the milk with staphylococci, and stimulated studies of the methods of production of the milk powder, and of methods for ensuring its safety.

The third important cause of food poisoning at the time was *Clostridium welchii* (now *Cl. perfringens*); *Cl. welchii* was first recognized as a food-poisoning bacterium in Birmingham during the war, but understanding of the disease was to a large extent the result of work in the Food Hygiene Laboratory (Hobbs *et al.*, 1953) which showed that, typically, the *Cl. welchii* food poisoning was attributable to the growth of the organism in cooked meat dishes allowed to cool slowly overnight.

Some pointers to future developments also appeared in the 1950s. There was an epidemic of typhoid fever, at Crowthorne, in which corned beef seemed to be implicated, but for which no convincing source was demonstrated (see p. 108). An outbreak of food poisoning due to the consumption of cockles was recorded but unresolved (see p. 146); there was interest in "winter vomiting disease" also unresolved but with the possible implication of bread (see p. 145), and there was preliminary evidence for the possible importance of fertilizers and animal feedstuffs as reservoirs for salmonellas (see p. 108).

The Food Hygiene Laboratory had a very active educational programme directed at catering staff and sanitary inspectors, and both the Ministry of Health and the Ministry of Agriculture, Fisheries and Food set up committees and issued reports on the hygiene of catering but, as the Chief Medical Officer noted in 1953, all efforts made towards reduction were still without noticeable effect.

Diarrhoea among newborn infants

The Chief Medical Officer's report for 1946 noted an unusual prevalence of diarrhoea among newborn infants in maternity hospitals, often with a high mortality, but with no specific bacterial cause recognized. The epidemics continued at a high level in 1947 and then gradually became less of a problem in succeeding years. Although the first suggestion that particular types of *Escherichia coli* might be responsible had been published by Adam as far back as 1920, and developed by Bray (1945), Joan Taylor, the director of the Salmonella Reference Laboratory, was alert to this possibility and during the next few years she and colleagues in other PHLS laboratories (as well as Danish workers) studied the antigenic structure of *E. coli* and amassed convincing evidence that particular serotypes were clearly associated with the disease and were presumably its cause, although the mechanism of pathogenesis was not discovered. From about 1953 typing sera to allow recognition of the more common enteropathogenic strains were available to PHLS laboratories and a number of epidemiological studies were published; Rogers in the Birmingham Children's Hospital was also a leader in this field, collaborating closely with Joan Taylor. There was good evidence that infected infants could act as vehicles for transfer of infection between hospitals, and presumptive evidence for transfer within the hospital by fomites and the hands and clothes of the staff, and by contaminated feeds (Taylor, 1960). After about 1950, serious epidemics became much more rare; the decline was presumably attributable to improved general care in maternity and children's hospitals, for certainly the researches of the 1950s did not reveal a specific preventive measure. Over the years the number of recognized enteropathogenic serotypes increased but it was not until the toxin controversy of the 1970s that real interest in *E. coli* diarrhoea revived.

Dysentery

The dysentery epidemic of the 1950s presented at least three odd features; the unexplained upsurge in notified cases from some 2090 in 1947 to nearly 49,000 in 1956; a change in the seasonal prevalence to the spring; and the fact that, almost uniquely, the number of isolations reported by the laboratories has consistently equalled about 90 per cent of the number of notifications received by medical officers of health. The final feature must presumably mean that practitioners notify only when they have specific bacteriological confirmation that the diarrhoea is due to dysentery bacilli, but even so the concordance is extraordinary. Considering the number of cases it is perhaps surprising that the epidemic did not cause more concern than it did although the Chief Medical Officer's reports give much detail on geographical distribution and the Ministry asked the PHLS to set up a subcommittee to study the epidemiology of the infection in 1951. This committee deliberated for some years without coming to any very firm conclusions, although Dr Irene Hutchinson, in the Southampton laboratory, reported some revealing studies of the extensive environmental contamination with *Shigella sonnei* in the toilets of primary schools. The committee's trial of phthalylsulphathiazole prophylaxis did not show much benefit. But the occurrence of large numbers of small outbreaks in schools and day nurseries certainly served to get the urban laboratories well known in their communities. Dr Mair Thomas later published a long series of studies based on the work of the Edmonton sub-laboratory (Thomas and Tillett, 1975). Colicine typing for *Sh. sonnei* was developed by Abbott and Shannon (1958) in the Manchester laboratory, but its application did not prove to be of great help in unravelling epidemiology owing to the great number of types in the community.

Whooping cough

The disappointing trials of a vaccine to protect children against whooping cough, carried out in the Oxford laboratory during the later war years, have been mentioned previously (p. 23). The contrast between the success reported from the United States and the failure in England prompted the Medical Research Council to set up some further trials with various vaccines, and Cockburn was recruited to the PHLS to arrange and supervise the trials from a base in the Central Public Health Laboratory. With enthusiastic support from Cruickshank and from Professor (later Sir Austin) Bradford Hill, together with some advice from Dr Pearl Kendrick of Michigan, USA, and the MRC Whooping Cough Immunization Committee, Cockburn organized a whole series of properly controlled, double-blind, trials, comparing various vaccines against placebos, and later against other vaccines. These were probably the first adequately controlled field trials of vaccines in Britain and are now accepted as classical examples of how to test a new prophylactic in circumstances where no established satisfactory material is available. In all, 8000 children were observed in the placebo-controlled trials and some 30,000 in the later trials comparing vaccines. In 1951 the MRC was able to report that protection rates of 70–80 per cent could be expected (MRC, 1951; see also Cockburn, 1955) but the introduction of a national vaccination programme was delayed by the observation, in further field trials, of large variations in the protective activity of the different vaccines available. Many PHLS laboratories were involved in the trials to the extent of attempting to cultivate *Bordetella pertussis* from swabs, preferably pernasal swabs (Cockburn and Holt, 1948) and in helping various concurrent studies of antibiotic treatment for whooping cough – most proving rather disappointing. The official national programme for pertussis immunization was not started until 1957 but, despite the cautious advice of the Ministry and the MRC prior to 1956, a good many local authorities had already been offering vaccination to infants; this, coupled with non-specific improvements in the clinical care of young infants with respiratory diseases, doubtless accounted for the fact that, by 1956, there were only 95 deaths from whooping cough, compared with 808 in 1946.

Diphtheria

For diphtheria the vaccination programme was well under way by 1946 and was pursued vigorously by the Ministry; despite the large reservoirs in continental Europe, the numbers of notifications and deaths declined steadily. With the decline in numbers it became practicable and useful to encourage detailed bacteriological examination of all patients and a search for carriers, especially "dangerous carriers", among their contacts; this was advocated in the Chief Medical Officer's reports for 1949 and 1953. PHLS laboratories reported 1195 isolations of *Corynebacterium diphtheriae* in 1948. The Epidemiological Research Laboratory organized extensive trials of new diphtheria prophylactics, particularly PTAP (purified toxoid, aluminium-phosphate-precipitated), a topic discussed at almost all Staff Committee meetings in 1948 and 1949, and finally reported in 1954 (PHLS, 1954). There were also collaborative investigations of penicillin treatment for carriers (PHLS, 1948) and on methods of laboratory diagnosis. But, by the end of the 1950s, this disease had been reduced to small islands of infection, manifested by sporadic cases or small outbreaks, each justifying quite a lot of routine work but not stimulating new investigations or innovative methods.

Scarlet fever

Scarlet fever, like diphtheria, smallpox and enteric fever, is one of those diseases that history had placed at the start of the Chief Medical Officer's annual report "On the state of the public health"; by 1956 it would almost certainly not have been there without history, and indeed in the 1956 report the Chief Medical Officer averred that scarlet fever might have reached its nadir (which it had not). Repeatedly over the next 10 years there was recognition of the anomaly that scarlet fever was notifiable whereas other infections, due as Griffith had shown to the same streptococci, were not. But notification has continued, as a "useful indicator", though not very clearly of what. The frequency of acute sore throat, the ease with which a throat swab can be examined for haemolytic steptococci, and the intellectual satisfaction gained from isolating them and attributing to them the cause of the sore throat, have all combined to maintain interest in haemolytic streptococcal infections. In the United States there was also continuing interest, due largely to the big war-time epidemics in the Armed Forces. In the PHLS the streptococci were fortunate to have, in W.R. Maxted, an investigator of very considerable ingenuity and persistence.

The war-time experience in the United States led to the recognition of the fact that some carriers of haemolytic streptococci are particularly apt to disperse the bacteria and to be a focus of continuing secondary cases, and also of the relation of throat infection with steptococci of Lancefield's Group A to acute rheumatic fever. It was evident that proper epidemiological investigation of outbreaks of infection required the identification of the serotype of the streptococci isolated. Thanks to the past interests of individuals in the PHLS laboratories at Cambridge, Oxford and Cardiff, it was possible to devolve some of the work from the Streptococcus Reference Laboratory at Colindale to provide a service all through the country; the Colindale laboratory prepared the typing sera and provided back-up advice. Streptococcal serotyping had been developed independently by F. Griffith in London and Rebecca Lancefield working at the Rockefeller Institute in New York. Griffith used a slide agglutination method relying, as is now known, very largely on the T antigen, while Lancefield used a precipitin method which depended on the M antigen. In the Streptococcus Reference Laboratory both methods were used and it was one of the challenges to, and achievements of, the laboratory over the next two or three decades to reconcile the two methods and to convince American colleagues that both were needed for full identification. This achievement was to a great extent Maxted's.

The numerous small outbreaks of streptococcal infection and scarlet fever around 1947 stimulated the Staff Committee to set up a subcommittee on streptococcal infections, which initiated some studies of the distribution of streptococci in the community, reviewed again by the Staff Committee in 1950 with the relation to rheumatic fever much in mind. By 1952 it had been shown, in the United States, that acute glomerulonephritis was often a sequel to throat infections with type 12 streptococci, which led to further studies on the distribution of such streptococci in England and Wales and work to confirm the American claims (Wilmers *et al.*, 1954; Holmes and Williams, 1954). At this time also, studies of impetigo revealed that the streptococci, and also the staphylococci, isolated from the skin lesions usually fell into serotypes different from those predominant in other infections (Parker *et al.*, 1955). Concurrently, American experience and our own was showing that acute nephritis can be a sequel to steptococcal skin infections; the importance of the differences between "throat" and "skin" streptococci become clear much later (p. 113).

Maxted's technical innovations during this period included the use of a *Streptomyces* enzyme for extracting the group antigen, of bacitracin discs for the quick identification of Group A streptococci, the characterization of the phages attacking haemolytic streptococci (which did not then prove to be useful for typing but reappeared on the scene some 30 years later, p. 153), and studies of the relation of the surface structures of streptococci to their serotype. The contributions of the area laboratories during the period consisted in revealing the frequency with which nasal carriers of steptococci could reasonably be regarded as "dangerous"; the Cambridge laboratory in particular started a number of studies of small outbreaks in its territory that were to be continued for 30 years, but which have unfortunately never been fully documented.

Poliomyelitis

The knowledge that poliomyelitis was very prevalent in the Far East, from where many servicemen were returning in 1945–6, had alerted the authorities to the possibility of an epidemic, and indeed the PHLS had made plans to examine normal individuals in

Britain for antibody to poliovirus, but the size of the 1947 outbreak certainly came as a surprise, for the 1946 incidence was actually below that of 1938. During 1947 a total of 7507 cases of poliomyelitis, in its various forms, were notified, with 766 deaths. The number of cases of bulbar poliomyelitis was striking and, because some query had been raised as to the true diagnosis, MacCallum in the Virus Reference Laboratory tested material from 11 fatal cases by inoculation of monkeys, which was the only diagnostic method available at the time; six of the 11 showed typical signs of poliomyelitis. The PHLS was also asked to collaborate with the Ministry's officers in an epidemiological study. Spicer (1959) analysed the incidence rates in relation to meteorological factors for the years 1947–56, which seemed to indicate that both temperature and relative humidity had some effect on incidence, but no mechanism for the relation could be identified.

The incidence of poliomyelitis fluctuated, but remained at a historically high level for several years; the Chief Medical Officer noted that the total number of cases in the three years 1947–9 exceeded that for the previous 20 years. In 1951 the Virus Reference Laboratory set up a very large study to seek poliovirus in sewage – as an indicator of the reservoirs in the population; 30 sewage sampling points were tested in each of 96 small towns and villages, with the use of the cotton swabs devised by Moore for seeking carriers of typhoid bacilli. Pools of fluid expressed from the swabs were inoculated into monkeys, but only four specimens yielded virus (Goffe *et al.*, 1960).

By 1952 progress had been made with tissue culture for the isolation of poliovirus and by 1955 a few PHLS laboratories were equipped for this work. A striking breakthrough had come with the demonstration by Tomlinson, working first in the Bradford and later in the London County Hall PHLS laboratories, that it was practicable to test for poliovirus in HeLa cell cultures in a routine bacteriological laboratory (Tomlinson and Mitchell, 1956). This work undoubtedly sparked off a great deal of interest in virus diagnosis generally in the area laboratories and within a year 20 of them were equipped to isolate poliovirus. In 1956 the Staff Committee heard that the PHLS laboratories had isolated the virus from 819 specimens – a dramatic change from the single isolation of 1946 or the six of 1947.

The risk of poliomyelitis following prophylactic injections of various sorts ("provocation polio") was studied by an MRC committee, chaired by Wilson, which had Cockburn as one of its secretaries. With the help of medical officers of health, details were obtained of any cases of poliomyelitis in which there was a history of prophylactic inoculation within 12 weeks prior to the onset of the illness. Cockburn and J. Knowelden (the other secretary) visited most of the areas from which reports were received to assemble detailed records. The study revealed that there did indeed appear to be an increased risk, and that as many as 13 per cent of paralytic cases in children under two years of age could have been causally related to inoculation (MRC, 1956).

The first field trials of the Salk vaccine were conducted by another MRC committee, with the Virus Reference Laboratory assisting in tests on preliminary batches of vaccine. After the Ministry's vaccination programme using the Salk vaccine was initiated in 1956 an additional responsibility fell on the Epidemiological Research Laboratory to keep a watch for possible vaccine-associated cases of poliomyelitis. The successful vaccination programme meant that there was no longer a risk of provoking poliomyelitis by diphtheria or pertussis vaccination.

The increase in the facilities for the isolation of virus from suspect cases also allowed further exploration of the problems of non-paralytic poliomyelitis. In 1951 the Virus Reference Laboratory isolated a Coxsackie virus from one patient, among eight investigated, in a cluster of cases of benign meningo-encephalitic illness in Coventry (Galpine and Macrae, 1953) and in his report for 1953 the Chief Medical Officer speculated on the possibility that some of the patients diagnosed as suffering from non-paralytic poliomyelitis might in fact be infected with Coxsackie viruses, as had been shown in the USA by Dalldorf. The 1956 report of the Chief Medical Officer returned to this problem, which was of particular concern as a source of confusion or dismay in the vaccination programme. In fact, the Virus Reference Laboratory had isolated strains of echovirus from a number of outbreaks of aseptic meningitis occurring in the autumn of 1955 (Boissard *et al.*, 1957).

Influenza

In 1946 influenza, like diphtheria, was known to be active in the devastated cities of continental Europe and there were fears for the importation of a serious epidemic to Britain; the post-war pandemic of 1918 was often in mind. An important function for the new Virus Reference Laboratory at Colindale was therefore to set up a diagnostic service, and this was available by the winter of 1946–7. Dr L. Hoyle (Figure 22), the

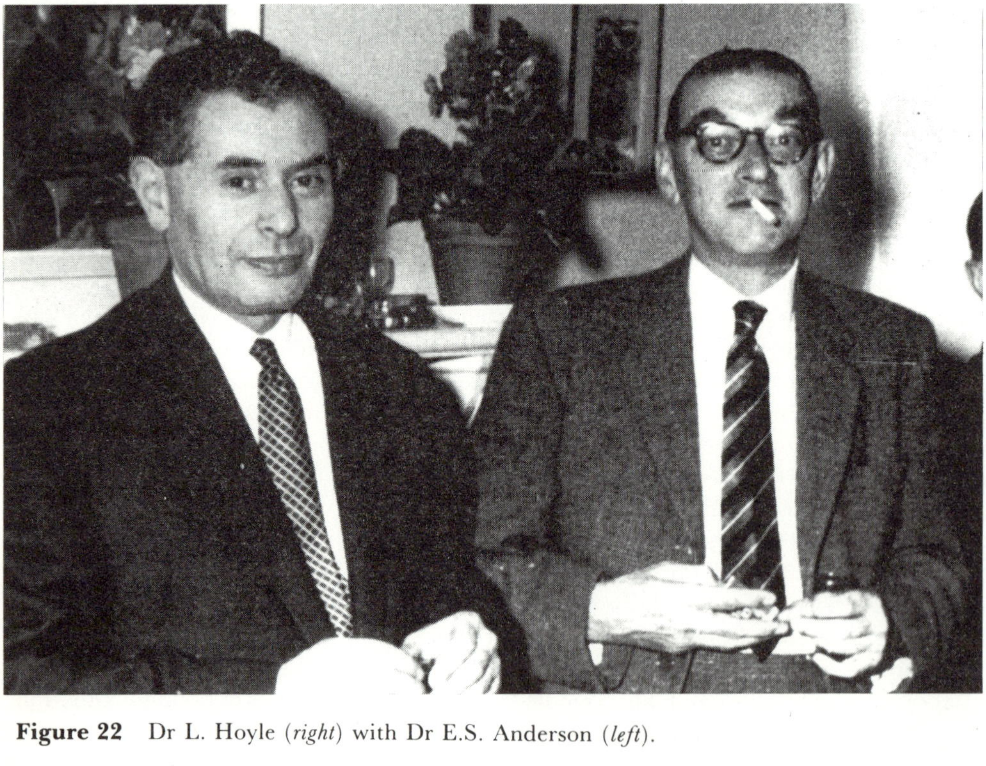

Figure 22 Dr L. Hoyle (*right*) with Dr E.S. Anderson (*left*).

director of the PHLS laboratory at Northampton, was already working on influenza, and in particular on the development of a diagnostic complement fixation test, and his laboratory, too, offered a serological diagnostic service. At this time the main epidemiological intelligence centre was at the National Institute for Medical Research, where the World Health Organization had set up the World Influenza Centre, under Dr C. H. Andrewes, in 1948.

Hoyle pursued a long series of very important researches, working largely on his own (and often almost totally enveloped in cigarette smoke) in the Northampton laboratory. He explored the growth cycle of the virus in hens' eggs, and described the intracellular phase of multiplication, suggesting that there was an intracellular multiplying form that differed from the extracellular form, and confounding those who then viewed viral multiplication as fission similar to bacterial. He later studied the relation of biological activity to the chemical structure of the virus and the release of the virus from the infected cell, showing that when the virus was released from the cell it was enclosed in an outer membrane derived from the cell wall. Hoyle was, during this period, one of the leading investigators in experimental virology (see Hoyle, 1952, 1954; Hoyle and Frisch-Niggemeyer, 1955).

By 1951, 10 PHLS laboratories were able to offer a serological diagnostic service; virus isolation, however, was available only at Colindale and Northampton (apart from the National Institute for Medical Research and Sheffield University). The considerable epidemic of 1951 indicated the need for a more rapid intelligence service, and the Chief Medical Officer noted that sick-absence claims, reported to the Ministry of Pensions and National Insurance, were utilized for this purpose for the first time. The Chief Medical Officer also mentioned general practitioner "spotters" and the data from the Registrar General – but not information from the diagnostic laboratories. In association with vaccine trials, most of which were sponsored by the MRC, an influenza spotting scheme was put into operation by the PHLS in 1954–5 in 17 large cities (increased to 19 to 1955–6). In each centre six local general practitioners were found who were willing to take blood samples during the acute and convalescent stages from suspect cases during the five winter months. Similar large surveys were conducted in the Royal Air Force. By 1954 the PHLS information was considered an integral part of the intelligence system, and indeed in 1955 the Chief Medical Officer commented on the important part played by the laboratories, in collaboration with the general practitioner "spotters" and the World Influenza Centre.

During the decade the MRC organized several trials of influenza vaccines, in which PHLS laboratories participated, though none was particularly encouraging.

Hepatitis

Hepatitis had been recognized as a serious problem during the war years, and had been made notifiable in the Ministry's Eastern Region; in 1943 the MRC had constituted a Jaundice Committee which organized a number of field and laboratory investigations between 1943 and 1947. A.M. MacFarlan was seconded from the EPHLS for the epidemiological studies, which defined the pattern of the disease and the incubation period. MacCallum, whose interest in hepatitis derived from his studies of the jaundice sometimes induced by yellow-fever vaccination (due to the human serum in the vaccine), attempted and failed to transmit the infection to a varied collection of animals, but demonstrated the transmission to human volunteers by the administration of faecal suspensions (MacCallum *et al.*, 1951).

In the early post-war years, Cockburn investigated the use of gamma-globulin and adult serum in the prevention of measles and demonstrated the effectiveness of the globulin (PHLS, 1950). In a subsequent trial of concentrated adult serum, Cockburn and his colleagues were unfortunate enough to witness a severe outbreak of hepatitis associated with one batch of the concentrated serum (Cockburn, Harrington *et al.*, 1951); gamma-globulin from the same batch produced hepatitis in only one of 58 recipients.

Measles, chickenpox and mumps

In the Epidemiological Research Unit at Cirencester, Dr Hope Simpson studied the spread of measles, chickenpox and mumps within the families in his general practice; he also demonstrated clearly an association of shingles with chickenpox (Simpson, 1954).

Q fever

Q fever was first recognized as occurring in Britain in a small outbreak of illness among the staff in a London hospital (MacCallum *et al.*, 1949). This was following by a number of surveys to determine the reservoirs in Britain, and it was eventually demonstrated that there were several areas in which cows and sheep were infected (Marmion and Stoker, 1958), a picture confirmed by the investigation of an outbreak in rural Wales in 1956 (Evans, 1956).

Venereal diseases

The reason for the lack of concern in PHLS planning with the venereal diseases has already been mentioned as stemming from the prior existence of a network of diagnostic laboratory services supported by local authorities (p. 3); indeed in 1946 the Staff Committee was told that tests for the diagnosis of venereal diseases would be within the province of the hospital pathologists, and (in 1947) that PHLS laboratories would have to claim a fee if they carried them out. However, the Ministry's venereal diseases laboratory had been transferred to the PHLS in 1946 and the director, Dr I.N. Orpwood Price, conducted investigations into the complement fixation tests and the Kahn test. In 1953 the laboratory commenced the study of the treponemal immobilization test (Wilkinson, 1954), which Orpwood Price's successor, A.E. Wilkinson, was to carry out for many years with a skill probably unmatched by anyone in the country.

Tuberculosis

Tuberculosis was, like the venereal diseases, an infection that was expected to fall within the province of the hospital pathologists, and although the Staff Committee held a number of technical discussions on laboratory diagnostic methods in 1948, 1952 and 1953, PHLS laboratories were not much concerned in innovation or epidemiological research. In 1953, however, Collins published the first of a series of studies on methods of distinguishing tubercle bacilli from various other related mycobacteria, and in 1954 Spicer published an important paper in which he applied the generation method of analysis to mortality trends from respiratory tuberculosis. Reference is made elsewhere (p. 76) to the growing realization that tuberculosis might be an occupational hazard for laboratory workers, and to the design of the first protective cabinet.

Hospital-acquired infections

During the decade to 1956 very few PHLS laboratories were carrying out routine bacteriology for general hospitals and although hospital-acquired infection had had some limited attention during the war years, it was not a topic of widespread concern until the mid-1950s. The only exceptions were in maternity units, where staphylococcal skin infections had been troublesome during the war and had been investigated in Cardiff (Allison and Hobbs, 1947), and the epidemic diarrhoea of the newborn referred to previously (p. 65). There were, of course, also examples of salmonella infections in hospitals.

However, the facilities for the phage typing of staphylococci offered to all hospital laboratories by the reference laboratory at Colindale were soon utilized to examine strains from a growing number of outbreaks of surgical wound infection and, from 1954 onwards, infections in maternity wards and among nursing staff. Analysis of these data revealed the existence of a number of staphylococci with characteristic phage types that were evidently producing epidemics in many hospitals and it was possible to document the rise in prevalence of the notorious "type 80/81" staphylococci as part of the world-wide pandemic (Williams, 1959). The PHLS laboratory in Middlesbrough, opened in 1951, was one of those carrying out routine hospital bacteriology and it was not long before Dr R. Blowers, the director, was invited to study an outbreak of surgical wound infection in a thoracic surgery unit. He traced the infections to the operating room (Blowers *et al.*, 1955) and thus started a whole series of important investigations into operating theatre ventilation, design and practice, and into hospital-acquired infection generally (see p. 112). Studies of maternity hospital infections with staphylococci were carried out in several laboratories; Jellard (1957), in the Plymouth laboratory, recognizing the importance of the infant's umbilical stump as a reservoir of infection, introduced routine umbilical disinfection. The fact that she used a violet dye as the disinfectant ensured that her method would not persist, but the innovation was followed in many places by the development of less glaring but equally effective agents.

Type identification was a requisite for the study of staphylococcal infections; phage typing proved an adequate though by no means ideal method and, despite Betty Hobbs' valiant efforts to make sense of serotyping, became the standard. Extensive tests in the Staphylococcus Reference Laboratory gave some indications of the reproducibility and precision of the method (Williams and Rippon, 1952). Phyllis Rountree, visiting the laboratory from Australia in 1948, studied the phenomenon of lysogenicity (Rountree, 1949) and initiated a series of investigations into the nature and behaviour of staphylococcal phages and their relation to phage type that were to continue in the hands of Joan Rippon and later Elizabeth Asheshov until the late 1970s. By 1956, 10 area laboratories were providing phage typing services, often used by hospitals in their neighbourhood; all the phage preparations were supplied from Colindale and periodic quality control trials were started in 1957.

The constitution of an Air Hygiene Unit within the Streptococcus and Staphylococcus Reference Laboratory has already been mentioned (p. 52). "Air hygiene" was a concept developed by W.F. Wells in Philadelphia in the 1930s after he had appreciated the fact that some of the microbe-carrying droplets dispersed from the mouth and nose in coughing, talking and sneezing can evaporate to "droplet nuclei" small enough to remain airborne for a considerable period and so travel some distance indoors. Wells described a method utilizing ultra-violet irradiation of the air, which he called "sanitary ventilation", by which he claimed to reduce the spread of measles and chickenpox in schools. The war-time work of Bourdillon, Lidwell and Lovelock, summarized in their massive MRC Special Report "Studies in air hygiene" (Bourdillon *et al.*, 1948) took up many of Wells's ideas and developed sophisticated instruments and a more sophisticated theory, but still with the idea that carriage in small airborne droplet nuclei was a most important route for the spread of pathogens entering by the respiratory tract. Techniques and ideas relevant to the spread of airborne pathogens were, of course, also developed during the war years in connection with bacteriological warfare, at the Ministry of Defence's Microbiological Research Department (later Establishment) at Porton Down, but these were never much utilized in studies of intramural spread.

Cruickshank became very interested in the subject of airborne infection and with his encouragement the Medical Research Council agreed to sponsor a field trial of ultra-violet air irradiation in six schools in the outer London borough of Southall. Under the MRC Air Hygiene Committee, I was responsible for developing the bacteriological monitoring of the trial; Lidwell, then based at the Common Cold Research Unit at Salisbury, was responsible for the instrumentation, and Donald D. Reid, of the London School of Hygiene and Tropical Medicine, took care of the statistics. Although the results were essentially negative, in that ultra-violet irradiation made very little difference to the spread of infection, the trial was valuable as a test-bed for developing air-sampling methods, which were to be the continuing theme of the Air Hygiene Unit, and to provide recurrent opportunities for Lidwell to display ingenuity and an ability to devise and build suitable instruments to tackle each successive problem. One particularly elegant example was his "pagoda" sampler for size-grading of airborne bacteria-carrying particles (Lidwell, 1959; see Figure 23). With this instrument he was able to show that the median equivalent diameter of airborne particles carrying staphylococci was around 14 μm, far larger than a droplet nucleus.

Apart from the ultra-violet trial, the Air Hygiene Unit investigated the bacterial content of the air in London underground trains, in boot and shoe factories in Northampton and Leicester, and in coal mines. Hexylresorcinol was tested as an air disinfectant in offices of the Ministry of Pensions and National Insurance in Newcastle, and had no detectable effect; from 1952 onwards the ventilation of hospital wards and

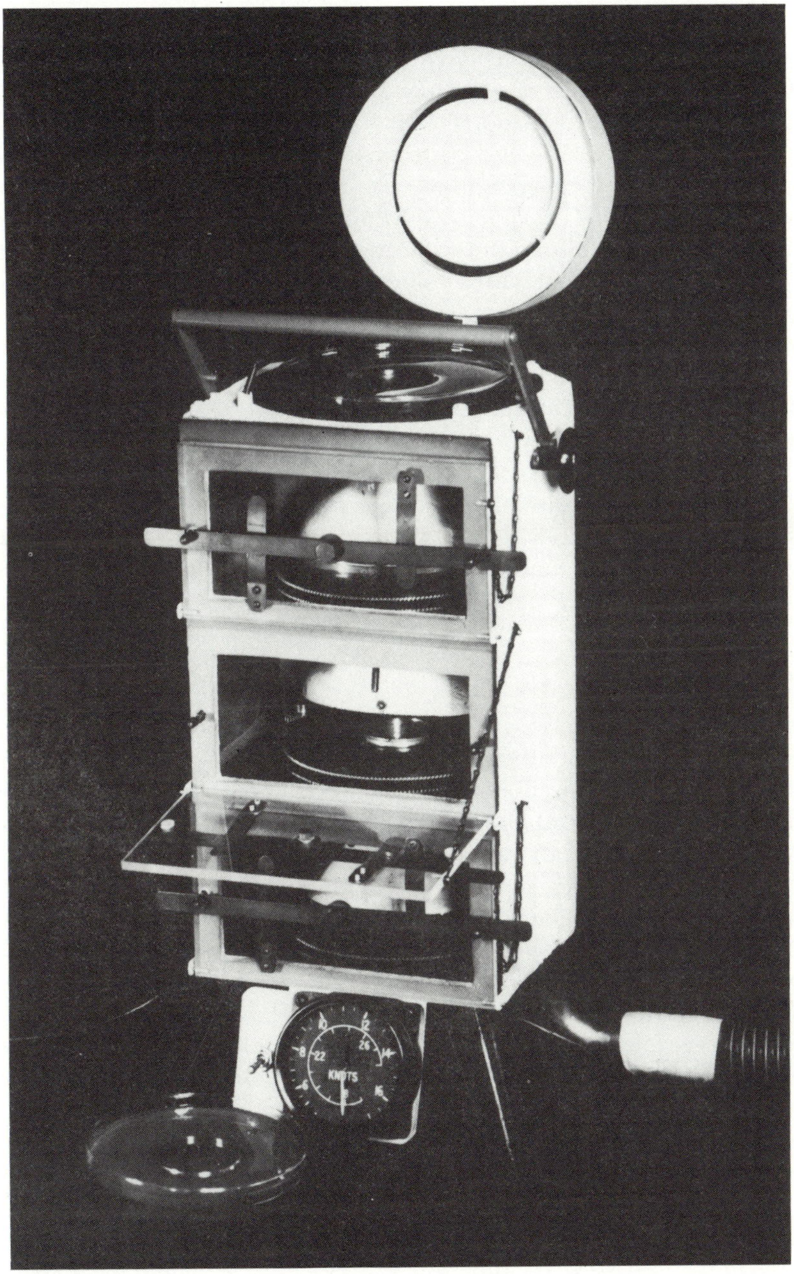

Figure 23 Lidwell's "pagoda" air-sampler.

operating theatres became a topic of increasing interest. Around 1956 the unit developed joint studies with Professor R.A. Shooter at St Bartholomew's Hospital which were to be very profitable for many years.

Disinfection of bedclothes, particularly blankets, became a fashionable topic in the early 1950s after it had been shown how heavily contaminated with staphylococci hospital blankets may become, and when it was appreciated how rarely the blankets were changed between successive patients. Various methods were proposed for disinfecting blankets, or for making them retain their contaminating bacteria rather than release them. The PHLS appointed a committee on formaldehyde disinfection, which was chaired by Wilson and worked to make the best of what is inevitably a rather bad job; it eventually came out with a voluminous report (PHLS, 1958*b*). Around the same time the Portsmouth laboratory was involved, with E.M. Darmady, in the development of a central sterile supply service, and methods for the dry-heat sterilization of syringes.

By 1956 the Chief Medical Officer was commenting that hospital infection was becoming a major interest of the bacteriological epidemiologist, and that there was a need to discover its real incidence. Two reasons were advanced to account for the increase: a decline in aseptic discipline and an increase in the use of antibiotics; perhaps increased virulence of the staphylococci was also relevant. PHLS laboratories became more and more involved in studies of incidence and of etiology during the next few years.

Laboratory safety

In the light of the recent eruptions of concern over laboratory safety, it is interesting to look back to the ideas in circulation in the 1940s and 1950s. The Staff Committee discussed the appropriate vaccinations for members of the staff at a 1947 meeting; in conformity with the tradition already established, directors were to have full discretion on the programme for their laboratories and at a further discussion in 1948 the same applied to tuberculin testing and chest radiography. But, in December 1948, the chairman reported on a fifth, fatal, case of typhoid fever contracted in a laboratory and indicated that the MRC was considering making vaccination against typhoid fever compulsory, with revaccination at 6–12 month intervals (as recommended by Felix).

In a Staff Committee discussion on tuberculosis in laboratory workers in 1949, the chairman wondered whether there was really any risk in the course of ordinary bacteriological activities. There had been nine cases of tuberculosis in PHLS staff in the past 10 years, but most of those infected had been exposed outside the laboratory. Nevertheless the Committee recommended tuberculin testing and chest X-rays for new entrants to the staff. In 1950 another fatal case of laboratory-acquired typhoid fever was reported. It was still thought difficult to judge claims on the prevalence of laboratory infection; on this occasion it was reported that there had been 11 cases of tuberculosis in the past 10 years and "a few" cases of typhoid and paratyphoid fever with evidence of laboratory origin. Directors were urged to keep records.

In 1954 the Staff Committee had an invitation from D.D. Reid, of the London School of Hygiene and Tropical Medicine, to participate in a trial to measure the incidence of tuberculosis in laboratory workers; the Committee's first reaction was unfavourable, envisaging various ethical, practical and statistical problems. However, after a few month's cogitation and on hearing that hospital laboratories were participating, the Committee agreed that the PHLS should take part. At the same meeting members were very critical of some wall-charts on safety measures prepared by the National Association for the Prevention of Tuberculosis and set up a working party to prepare some PHLS advice. The working party soon found that the problem was bigger than had been thought and stimulated some research into the excretion of tubercle bacilli in the urine of infected guinea-pigs (being used in quite large numbers in the testing of milk and some clinical specimens) and into protective cabinets. Tomlinson reported his observation that the opening of screw-capped bottles could generate an aerosol (Tomlinson, 1957) and in December 1955 the prototype PHLS safety cabinet (Williams and Lidwell, 1957) was demonstrated at a technical discussion on protective measures against laboratory infection with tuberculosis. The meeting also had a report from the working party detailing several recommendations, eventually incorporated in the PHLS report (PHLS, 1958*c*). By October 1956 Reid was able to give a report on his now classical survey (Reid, 1957), which demonstrated an excess of tuberculosis in laboratory workers. Argument on the need for vaccination against typhoid fever grumbled on and, ironically, at the meeting when Felix's death was recorded, the Committee took the first firm steps to softening the rules for the very frequent revaccination that Felix had always held to be essential.

Food, water and environmental specimens

In 1955, the first year for which detailed records are available, PHLS laboratories received 361,000 requests for the examination of food, water and other environmental specimens. The development of methods and the devising of standards was a major preoccupation for the Staff Committee and the subcommittees that it set up (see Appendix Table 8). The energetic activities of the subcommittee on the bacteriological standards for ice-cream has already been mentioned, while another long-running show was the subcommittee on bacteriological standards for drinking water, set up to assist in the revision of the Ministry of Health Report No. 71 on the same topic; the revision was published in 1956.

One committee whose report, published in 1959 (PHLS, 1959*a*), proved distinctly controversial was that on the sewage contamination of bathing beaches. The committee made bacteriological studies over five years of more than 40 popular bathing beaches around the coasts of England and Wales. It also made a special inquiry, through the local medical officers of health, of all notified cases of enteric fever occurring in coastal areas, which identified just four cases of paratyphoid fever apparently associated with bathing in what were recognized as highly polluted beaches. On behalf of the committee, Cockburn and Dr W.S. Parker, the medical officer of health of Brighton, made a similar inquiry into all cases of the poliomyelitis notified from coastal areas, as well as a series of matched controls; no evidence could be found of an association of poliomyelitis with sea bathing. It was concluded that, despite the fact that many beaches were obviously heavily polluted with sewage, the pollution, though aesthetically very unpleasant, constituted a negligible health hazard. In its determination to be scientifically unassailable on the health hazards, the report perhaps underplayed the aesthetics and the likely emotional impact of a report that concluded that "the great majority of beaches studied were subject to contamination with sewage". The public reaction had not moved far from the point made by Wade Frost in 1916. "In the former days," he wrote, "when there was a widespread belief that epidemics of disease were caused by foul-smelling gases, the offensive conditions in a highly polluted stream were considered a gross menace to the health of persons in the immediate vicinity . . .". He added that "Nowadays . . . it is for the sake of common decency rather than for the prevention of the specific fevers . . ." that these nuisances should be abated.

The bacteriological control of milk supplies was also a perennial topic; a long series of collaborative investigations and frequent discussions eventually led to the adoption of the Aschaffenburg–Mullen test in place of the Kay–Graham test for checking the pasteurization of milk, and to the validation of the ring test for detecting brucella organisms in milk (PHLS, 1956*a*, *b*). Mr Peel, the head technician in the Bradford laboratory, was particularly active in collaboration with the sanitary inspectors in the pursuit of studies on brucellosis, as was Dr D.J.H. Payne, at Northallerton.

Other related topics of study included the bacterial contamination of meat in slaughterhouses and of water in swimming pools, the cleaning of infant-feeding bottles, the bacteriological grading of shellfish, and the bacteriological examination of water-works employees. One committee devised a modified methylene blue test for the grading of fresh cream.

Administrative Reorganization: Creation of the Statutory Public Health Laboratory Service Board

Although the Medical Research Council had, in 1952, agreed to the indefinite continuation of its administration of the Service, it was not long before doubts were raised. It seems that it was Himsworth, the Secretary of the Council, who first became concerned that the PHLS staff could receive substantially greater salaries than those paid to the Council's own research staff. This difference was in part simply due to the fact that National Health Service salary scales were higher than the university scales to which the MRC was tied. But there were two other factors. The PHLS staff were eligible for "distinction awards"; this added to the possible discrepancy, compared with MRC research staff, who, in general, were not. Since such awards were related to clinical responsibility there was also a risk that senior staff with heavy administrative duties might receive a smaller award than more junior staff largely engaged in clinically related work; this system was clearly unsatisfactory for a heirarchical service such as the PHLS. Moreover, it seemed to the MRC that not all the PHLS staff promoted to the consultant grade had achievements comparable to those required for promotion to senior posts on the research staff.

Accordingly, in 1954, it was decided to explore with the Ministry some alternative administrative arrangements for the PHLS that would preserve its ability to operate nation-wide with central control, and with as much of its traditional elasticity of management as possible.

Various models were discussed, including transfer of financial responsibility to the Ministry with the MRC retaining scientific direction, or retention of the MRC administration with a radical restructuring of the PHLS salary scales, on a hierarchical basis, which would have meant substantial salary reductions for some; because it was accepted that these could not be imposed on those in post, it was suggested that the lower scales should apply only to new entrants (implying the maintenance of inequitable differentials for up to 30 years!). It was finally agreed, however, that Council could not renege on its 1949 agreement that medical salaries in the PHLS should be equated to those in the National Health Service, and the discussions through 1954 and 1955 focused on a plan by which the Ministry of Health would itself assume overall administrative responsibility for the Service, and would be the employer, at least for all the medical and other senior staff. The Ministry would also run the reference laboratories; the appointment of junior staff in area and regional laboratories might be delegated to the respective Board of Governors or Hospital Management Committee in whose premises the laboratory was sited, although the relation of these laboratories to the central administration of the PHLS does not appear to have been spelt out. The

Ministry was to be assisted by a small advisory committee comprising the Chief Medical Officer (in the chair), two representatives of the MRC, one medical and one administrative officer of the Ministry, one member from the field of preventive medicine, and one from academic bacteriology.

Up to this point the PHLS staff had heard little but rumours. Landsborough Thomson attended a Staff Committee meeting in June 1955. He described the Council's difficulties, stressed the Council's concern to preserve the integrity of the Service, and said that for some time it had been clear to him that there would be a need to "retreat strategically to a carefully prepared position". The first stage had been the establishment of the PHLS Board within the MRC structure; the next must be to give the Board some autonomous position, and long discussions were in progress with the Ministry to this end. It was certainly Landsborough Thomson's continuing hope that if the PHLS Board could not remain part of the MRC, it should be given independent status somehow; he favoured incorporation under the Companies Act.

Nevertheless, despite Landsborough Thomson's assertions at the June Staff Committee meeting and despite reservations expressed in the Council by E.T.C. Spooner (who had been on the staff of the EPHLS), the MRC agreed on 22 July that the Ministry's plan should be accepted, subject to detailed negotiations on staff, buildings and finance. At a Staff Committee meeting in October 1955, Wilson informed the directors that the Service was to come under the direct administration of the Ministry, possibly from 1 April 1956. Although the detailed administrative structure was not yet known (surely he cannot have been so naive as to believe that it could all be settled in six months?), the directors were told not to be too alarmed! Needless to say, the Ministry's officers, in a letter to the MRC dated 19 October, required a very great deal of detailed information on staff (even including cleaners), on buildings, and on supply of materials. The date for the transfer to the Ministry was postponed to 1 October 1956.

It is very difficult to see how these proposals ever reached the advanced state of planning that they did; whether there were some in the Ministry who wished to gain control of the Service, or whether it was simply a reluctance to consider the creation of a new structure to meet the special requirements of the situation, is not apparent. In any case, in the summer of 1956 the Treasury entered the debate and it soon became clear that the proposed integration of the PHLS into the Ministry was not viable. The Treasury pointed out that such integration would create a new but equally embarassing salary discrepancy within the Ministry, that the integration would appear to increase by about 1000 the numbers in the Civil Service, that the work was not of a nature appropriate to a government department, that the proposal would certainly be unpopular with the staff of the Service, and that it would probably cause concern in the medical profession generally and in particular in the universities with public health laboratories attached.

The Ministry's plan was dead, and the MRC had to agree to continue its administrative role, first until April 1958, and then October 1958, and then October 1959. The death of the Ministry's plan was followed by a period of astoundingly long-drawn correspondence and discussion – long-drawn not because of its volume but because of the intervals between successive items. The Treasury would have preferred the retention of the status quo, but the MRC was insistent that it could not bear the continuing embarrassment of the salary differentials. In addition it regarded as unsatisfactory the arrangement by which it had the responsibility for running the Service while so many of the important policy decisions were reserved to the Ministry. The delegation to the PHLS Board also meant that the Council itself was contributing little but name, and not deriving any great benefit. It was time, they said, for the PHLS to flee the nest.

By April 1957 it seems to have been tacitly agreed that the establishment of an independent PHLS Board was the solution, and after a further year's delay the conclusion had been reached that the only practicable solution was to create, by legislation, an independent board within the National Health Service, similar to a regional hospital board. Quite suddenly it was found that parliamentary time could be made available. The proposal agreed in the autumn of 1958 was that the reconstituted board would employ the staff (who would therefore not become civil servants) and run the Service. It was originally envisaged that the Chairman of the Board should be the Chief Medical Officer of the Ministry – perhaps the last vestige of the plan for integrating the PHLS into the Ministry – but that the nine members of the board would be representatives of the MRC, professional bacteriologists, medical officers of health and medical administrators. It was proposed that the administrative staff of the board should be civil servants seconded from the Ministry, although this was later modified so that some, including the very important post of Secretary to the Board, could be seconded from the MRC, so as to preserve continuity. The Public Health Laboratory Service Bill, based on these proposals, had its first reading in the House of Lords on 9 December 1959.

In January 1960, Landsborough Thomson again attended a meeting of the Staff Committee – nearly five years after he had come to a meeting to tell the directors that the MRC could not continue its administration of the Service – and explained that the only way to get a national PHLS had been to limit its activities to public health bacteriology. Although, with the development of closer collaboration with hospital laboratories, he could foresee the possibility of a national bacteriological service, the PHLS Bill which had in the end taken shape at rather short notice was drawn up to provide a maximum of continuity with the existing structure.

The Bill was discussed by the Staff Committee and one clause that gave rise to some concern was the rather rigid definition of the membership of the board, and the omission of any representative of the hospital service. Incidentally it was explained that a suggestion to use the word "microbiological" in place of "bacteriological" had been rejected because it was feared that this might be thought to be widening the scope of the Service beyond that which had been prescribed in the original National Health Service Act.

The Bill received the Royal Assent on 29 July 1960 and the Minister issued an Order bringing the Act into force on 1 August 1961. The MRC had, therefore, yet again to postpone its handover to that date, some seven years after it had initiated discussions for the change of administration.

Thus the "[provision] of a bacteriological service . . . for the control of infectious diseases" envisaged in the National Health Service Act of 1946 was now delegated to a statutorily established board to operate in parallel with the regional boards administering the hospitals and the hospital microbiology laboratories. The principle that public health microbiology had requirements different from those called for in hospital work had been accepted. The chief difference stemmed from the fact that infectious diseases commonly ignore administrative boundaries and were held to require a national service for their control. But already, by 1960, 25 of the 60 PHLS laboratories were in fact providing clinical bacteriological services for the hospitals in which they were situated, and this proportion was destined to grow. The challenge of the next 20 years was to find ways to reconcile the requirement for laboratories to become involved in the first-line diagnostic work for general hospitals, where many of the problems of infectious disease were to be found, with the wider requirements for the support of the community public health services, and the provision of nation-wide epidemiological support. The first meeting of the statutory Board had one paper which contained the phrase "since the PHLS is part of the NHS . . ."; this assertion cannot be justified by any explicit statement in the legislation, and the absence of such a statement has been the basis of a number of the problems that have arisen in subsequent years.

Until 1961 the PHLS administration had naturally been within the MRC offices, latterly at 26 Old Queen Street, Westminster. The MRC purchased new accommodation in Park Crescent, on the edge of Regent's Park, for its headquarters in 1961, and the PHLS was able to rent a suite of rooms there, to which its headquarters office moved in July 1961. Mr D.V.T. Fairrie was seconded from the MRC staff to the post of Secretary to the Board – the chief executive officer – and proceeded to assemble a team of administrative officers, some on secondment from the Ministry of Health, preserving as much of the MRC philosophy of organization as possible and ensuring an approach rather different from that adopted in the National Health Service.

The statutory Public Health Laboratory Service Board met for the first time on 16 June 1961, with Landsborough Thomson in the chair, and the Director of the Service "in attendance". The membership of the Board is given in Appendix Table 7.

The Second Phase: 1957–69

The previous chapters brought the account of the work of the Service up to 1956. A second convenient division seems to be from 1957 to 1969, covering the period when the Service expanded to its greatest complement of laboratories and ending when a plan for reduction and some rationalization had been accepted, and at a time when the rebuilding of the Central Public Health Laboratory at Colindale had been agreed. Epidemiologically, the period saw the "conquest" of poliomyelitis, the reduction to a trickle of cases of diphtheria, the last imported cases of smallpox (apart from one in 1973), the virtual eradication of bovine tuberculosis and the initiation of a brucellosis eradication programme, the uncovering of various new reservoirs of foodborne infection and food poisoning, and the first recognition of the exotic viral haemorrhagic fevers in Europe.

It was in the period from 1957 to 1969 that the PHLS evolved from being a service parallel and complementary to the hospital pathology service to one that was, *de facto*, more and more an integral part of it, although the implications of this change were never defined in a formal way.

Relations with the hospital pathology service

The debate on the extent to which PHLS laboratories should be involved in hospital work was a recurrent topic at the Staff Committee and to a lesser extent at the PHLS Board meetings during the period. In September 1957 the "functions of the PHLS" formed the topic of a Staff Committee discussion. Some members stressed the need, in the light of the changed epidemiological situation since the start of the Service, for more formal links with general hospitals, because that was where the patients with infections were to be found, and they considered it perfectly possible to combine hospital and public health bacteriology in one laboratory. Others feared that such links would prejudice the cherished independence of the PHLS. Some thought that another alternative would be closer alignment with public health services generally, even with non-microbiological activities, or the industrial health services. All agreed on the importance of continuing research. Wilson was categorically opposed to venturing into public health outside microbiology (which would in any case have required legislation) and encouraged directors to work with the hospital services, while emphasizing that all PHLS work needed to be of use to the "public health". An anonymous "provincial pathologist", writing in *The Lancet* (Anon., 1958), saw the need for fitting the PHLS laboratories into the hospital laboratories along some integrated design.

In 1961 the newly constituted PHLS Board was given a paper on the "scope of the PHLS", in which it was stated that "the Service does not undertake work that is rightly within the province of the hospital or clinical pathologist, but is ready to help if other facilities are not available"; and it noted that an increasing number of laboratories were actually undertaking responsibility for hospital bacteriology under special arrangements. It mentioned the existence of many "joint laboratories" to which the hospital services contributed technical assistance (see p. 32). Later in 1961 another Board paper stated that while the requirements of the public health authorities must have priority, hospital bacteriology was also part of the Service's function, and its growing importance had to be recognized. In April 1962 the Board received an analysis of the work of the laboratories which showed only seven to be concerned purely with public and general practitioner work, 23 to do public health work together with some specified hospital work, such as venereal disease serology, and 29 to be in some ways joint laboratories with hospitals.

In 1962 the Medical Services Review Committee (Report, 1962) had suggested a merger of the PHLS with the hospital bacteriological service; in a Staff Committee discussion, Wilson "could not think that the Ministry would go back on a 20-year policy; the necessity for two separate services had been made plain by now". Nevertheless at the next meeting he is reported as expressing the hope that ultimately, by one means or another, the PHLS would become responsible for the bacteriology of the whole country!

The PHLS Annual Reports for 1963 and 1964 record increasing amounts of hospital work coming to the laboratories. The Board returned to the topic in January 1964, by which time James Howie had succeeded Wilson as director. Howie presented a paper, based on discussions at the Ministry, in which it had been agreed that, while the PHLS should not develop as the sole authority for providing bacteriological services for the National Health Service, where conditions were favourable collaboration "could go so far that one joint laboratory will undertake both public health and hospital bacteriology". Hospital bacteriology could be done by PHLS laboratories, under suitable arrangements, negotiated for each case, negotiations that were to include arrangements for the PHLS to recoup the full cost of the routine services provided for the hospital, epidemiology and virology being exempted from this reimbursement.

Early in 1965 Howie presented to the Staff Committee the text of a paper that he gave at a meeting of the Royal Medico-Chirurgical Society in Glasgow (Howie, 1965*a*). In this paper he asserted that the PHLS was an integral part of the National Health Service and that, though an increasing number of laboratories were doing routine bacteriology for hospitals, the hospital service had no need to fear a "take-over" by the PHLS: "Any mistaken notion that the PHLS aspires to be the sole provider of bacteriological services everywhere should be quickly forgotten". And, in reply to a letter in *The Lancet* from Edgar (1965), who had expressed dismay as "the bacteriology of one hospital after another is taken irreversibly into the PHLS", Howie (1965*b*) wrote that the PHLS would enter into a joint arrangement with a hospital only if invited to do so. At the same time he made it clear to directors that the PHLS needed always to justify its existence by its service to the community, both in epidemiology and in research. Moreover, the Service needed to educate its clients into the best use of the facilities available. Howie evidently felt that some laboratories – perhaps in consequence of the years of indecision – were less active than they should be, and inclined to lean too heavily on past reputation.

A formula for sharing the cost of joint laboratories with the hospital authorities was put to the Board in early 1966; it still relied on a division of the various headings of expenditure and allocation of the responsibility for meeting them either to the PHLS or to the hospital. It was thought that a division of two-thirds to the PHLS and one-third to the hospital would be generally appropriate.

The fears in the hospitals of the supposed predatory nature of the PHLS emerged again in 1967, when the PHLS set up regional centres for tuberculosis bacteriology, which offered to carry out antibiotic susceptibility tests on strains of tubercle bacilli for any hospital laboratories that wished it. Howie had to reassure one correspondent that the PHLS did not intend to take over all such work (although, indeed, it was the hope that as much of the work as possible would be concentrated in specialist laboratories, both to yield more accurate results and to reduce the number of staff exposed to the health hazards associated with performing the tests).

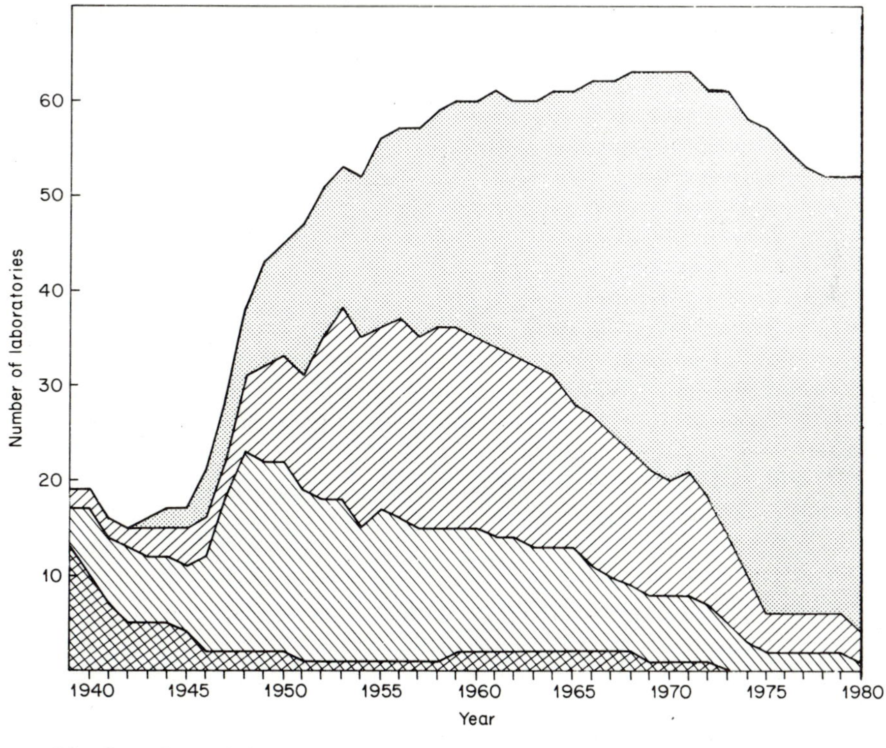

Figure 24 Constituent laboratories of the EPHLS and the PHLS, 1939–80: changes in location and function. ▭, in general hospitals, doing general hospital bacteriology; ▨, in hospitals but not doing general hospital bacteriology; ▧, not in hospitals, doing public health bacteriology only; ⊠, in schools and universities, doing public health bacteriology only.

By 1968 concern was being expressed that there was a risk of hospital work becoming so substantial and demanding that it would leave inadequate time or resources for "proper" public health work. At the same time it was recognized that recruitment of young medical graduates was likely to suffer if they were denied the direct access to patients that had become a normal part of the hospital medical microbiologist's work. The concern is, however, in interesting contrast to the concern expressed in 1955, that the development of the hospital pathology services would deprive the PHLS laboratories of work: clearly the PHLS had noted the advice – if you cannot beat them, join them.

In any case, during the 13-year period from 1957 to 1969 the development, often occurring opportunistically and generally somewhat in advance of the Board's appreciation of the fact, was clearly towards a Service composed of joint public health/hospital laboratories. During this period eight new constituent laboratories were opened, two of them replacing two of the three laboratories that were closed. Nine laboratories moved to new premises in general hospitals. Of the 59 constituent laboratories open in 1958, 23 were in general hospital premises and providing general bacteriological services to the hospitals; 21 were in hospitals, often infectious disease hospitals, but were not providing a full bacteriological service, and 15 were in public health departments or other premises away from hospitals and doing virtually only public health and general practitioner bacteriological work. By 1969, the corresponding figures for the 63 constituent laboratories were 42, 13 and eight (Figure 24). A reservation applying to all these figures is that, even when not responsible for the general bacteriological services of hospitals, PHLS laboratories were often performing some of the work, e.g. examining faecal specimens. An increasing number were also

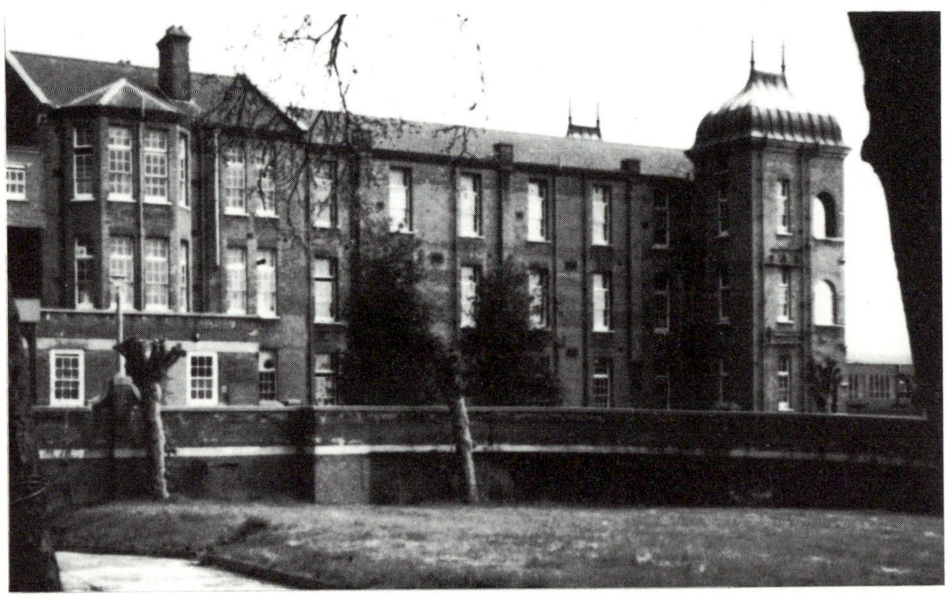

Figure 25 Whipps Cross Public Health Laboratory, London: this laboratory, in a converted ward, was opened in 1970.

offering some specialist services, especially virology or type identification of staphylococci or streptococci.

Of the new constituent laboratories, four were in new purpose-built structures, all except Bristol in hospital grounds; the others were in adapted accommodation (Figure 25). Of the nine moving to general hospitals, seven were in purpose-built units, but none of them was in the earlier tradition of a free-standing public health laboratory in the hospital grounds.

Administration and direction

In its last three years of life, the MRC Board seems to have been concerned solely with routine matters; no discussions on the future administration of the Service are recorded in its minutes. The statutory PHLS Board, which started work in 1961, soon decided that the tradition of managing with a minimum structure should be maintained: it decided at its first meeting that there was no need for a deputy chairman, treasurer or finance committee, though at a later 1961 meeting it did constitute an Estimates Committee (which persisted as the only finance committee of the Board until 1982). Although the papers recording the activities of the new PHLS Board are rather more detailed than those of its predecessor, the Board as such was only marginally more active; the policy of the Service was still very largely determined by the Director.

The Ministry had asked that the terms and conditions of service of the staff should be brought into line with those of the National Health Services and the Board spent some time considering what departures from those terms were called for. It secured Ministry permission to require senior medical appointments to be whole-time, to retain as a career post, with the possibility of promotion, the "senior bacteriologist" grade (equivalent to the National Health Service grade of senior hospital medical officer), and to include in consultants' contracts their liability to be moved from one laboratory to another at the Board's discretion. This last condition became something of a bogey that was held up by outsiders as an indication of the dictatorial style of management of the PHLS. In fact, I do not believe that it was ever used dictatorially; indeed it had the great advantage that consultants could move without having to be subjected to a new appointments committee, and could have their removal expenses paid. The Board had, at the same time, to concede that all new consultant appointments should be advertised publicly and filled on the recommendation of an Advisory Appointments Committee, constituted similarly to that for a hospital consultant. In his "Historical notes . . .", Wilson remarks that this change seriously curtailed the Director's freedom in making appointments and transfers; it ended the possibility that he could strike a bargain with a member of staff that if, say, he accepted an "unpopular laboratory in the North of England he would be brought down to fill a vacant post in the South in a few years' time"! Nevertheless, as Wilson admitted, the change to formal selection committees was one that had to come and, with the growing involvement in hospital work, it brought the enormous benefit of involving the hospital staff and authorities in the appointment of their potential colleagues; in this respect it can have done nothing but good.

Under the terms of the agreement following the 1961 Act, the Ministry had reserved the right to determine staff numbers. One of the Board's first activities was to consider an analysis of the medical staff structure and secure an increase in the number of consultant posts; in 1963 it was to request a substantial increase in the numbers of non-medical staff. Around the same time it considered the desirability of the PHLS being formally within the Ministry's Whitley Council machinery for negotiation on salaries and conditions of service, although it seems that no formal request to this effect was made, and no further mention can be found for some years. The fact that the PHLS, though required to conform to Whitley Council conditions, was not technically within the system was much later to be a serious bone of contention with the trade union representing some of the non-medical staff (p. 124).

The Board had also very soon to consider the appointment of a successor to G.S. Wilson – Sir Graham in the New Year's Honours List of 1962. After various inquiries Professor J.W. Howie, who held the chair of bacteriology in Glasgow, accepted the Board's invitation and took up the post on 1 October 1963. Wilson retired after 22 years as Director of the Service, and very fortunately spent part of the next year writing the "Historical notes . . ." on which the earlier part of my own account has leant heavily.

Whoever was responsible for the idea of the Service in the first place, there is no doubt of the magnitude of Wilson's achievement in bringing it to the position of renown and respect that it had gained by 1963. So far as leadership was concerned he had done this alone; he had no confidant other than Landsborough Thomson, he rarely engaged in a real consultative dialogue with members of the staff and he was distinctly reluctant to divulge his plans, so much so that Fairrie, who as the Board's chief executive officer had to make the necessary provision of resources, was not always clear what would be called for next. The load that Wilson carried was staggering and it was, and is, a mystery how he accomplished so much. His "Historical notes . . ." end with his own account of his duties. They reveal the magnitude of his activity, though not the means by which it could be achieved, but as they seem to offer an appropriate retrospect of Wilson's contribution, they may be reproduced almost in full.

> "One of the duties which the first Director [of the peace-time PHLS, cf. p. 15] always took seriously was the regular visitation of the laboratories. It was his aim to visit each of the provincial laboratories at least once a year and Colindale once a fortnight. In this way it was possible for him to gain a general impression of how well the laboratory was running, how satisfied the director and the staff were with their conditions of work . . . . Personal contact with the director and his staff, including the chief technician, and acquaintance of the exact location and working conditions of each laboratory, gave the Director of the Service a conspectus of the organization under his charge that he could not have gained in any other way and that proved immensely helpful to him in maintaining the loyalty of the staff . . . .
>
> "Another important function of the Director was the choice of sites for new laboratories and the size and design of the new buildings. When a private architect was employed, the Director always prepared, himself, ¼-inch drawings of the interior of the laboratory, putting in the fenestration, the lighting, the heating, the fixtures . . . .
>
> "Besides encouraging individual members to undertake research and sometimes suggesting problems for them, the Director often drew up plans for investigation on a larger scale, such as by a Working Party. Plans of this sort were usually discussed by the Staff Committee . . . . In this way the Director was able to promote investigation on a

large number of different problems and to arrange for the carrying out of field trials . . . .

"The Director was a member and occasionally chairman of numerous committees set up by such bodies as the Medical Research Council, the Ministry of Health, the Army Medical Department, the Agricultural Research Council, the British Medical Association, the Society of Medical Officers of Health or the World Health Organization . . . and he served as a liaison officer on other committees . . . so as to keep in touch with those working in the local authority and hospital fields.

"Though he did not insist on it, the Director liked to see every paper written by a member of the staff before it was sent for publication in a scientific journal. His purpose in this was to see that the paper was properly constructed; that it was written in unambiguous language; and that it was not likely to give offence to another scientific worker or to embarrass a government department . . . . In addition the Director usually checked all the numerical calculations himself and made certain that the references in the text agreed with those in the bibliography at the end of the paper . . . .

"Besides serving as an editorial adviser to the *Journal of Hygiene*, the Director, aided by his secretary, Miss Madeleine Barry, was responsible for editing Section II of the *Monthly Bulletin of the Ministry of Health and Public Health Laboratory Service* . . . .

"In addition to his official duties, the Director found himself consulted as an expert on a great variety of subjects . . . .

"During the war years, Professor Wilson was engaged part of his time in research . . . but after 1945 the demands of the Service . . . and of the Bacteriological Department of the London School of Hygiene and Tropical Medicine which had to be restarted and which required his attention until he was able to resign his professorship in 1947, precluded him from further work in the laboratory.

"Lastly, in his private capacity he had to devote some part of his time almost every day to keeping Topley and Wilson's 'Principles of Bacteriology and Immunity' up to date . . . .

"During the war years, after Dr Scott's death, Professor Wilson acted in a dual capacity, directing the public health laboratory at Oxford and the EPHLS as a whole from London. Though, when the war was over, he might have established his headquarters at Colindale, he preferred to work in the head office of the Medical Research Council . . . . The main reasons for this were (a) he found it convenient to be housed in the same building as the officers who were responsible for the general administration of the PHLS . . . ; (b) he did not want Colindale to be regarded as superior to the other laboratories in the Service . . . ; (c) there was far less chance of leakage of confidential information at the MRC headquarters than there would have been at Colindale; and members of the Service who wanted to see him privately could do so without attracting . . . attention . . . .

"The danger of leakage of information was one of the reasons why Professor Wilson never asked for a deputy. There would not have been sufficient work to keep a deputy fully occupied, so that, if one had been appointed he would have had to work part-time at Colindale. This would have created conditions which it seemed best to avoid . . . . Professor Wilson did his best to relieve the scientific staff of administrative duties in order that they might devote their time to the technical advancement of the Service. Had there not been such a shortage of bacteriologists, had the Treasury not placed such restrictions on manpower, and had the office accommodation been less cramped, the Director's decision not to ask for a deputy might well have been different.

"In conclusion, it may be said that the Director's method of administration was essentially a personal one. Though remaining detached and perhaps somewhat aloof, he was yet familiar with the personal history and background of every scientific member of the staff and was often able to deal helpfully with situations in a way that would have been impossible under a bureaucratic system."

As a gloss on this autobiographical note I might add two illustrative anecdotes. On one of his fortnightly visits to my laboratory at Colindale we had come round by some route that I cannot recall to the topic of carpentry. Wilson told me of his interest in woodworking and of some of the jobs that he had in hand; as he left he added "but only on Saturday, Williams". And Madeleine Barry recalled that if she visited Wilson's home on a Saturday afternoon, Wilson would have worked out all that needed to be done in the garden, and always had a reserve programme of jobs that could be done under cover in case of rain. She said that Wilson achieved all he did by planning and by taking care to avoid doing anything that was not absolutely necessary. The bicycling, which might be thought to fall into the latter category, must have been one of the rare actions that he deliberately undertook to give him time to think and to "recharge his batteries".

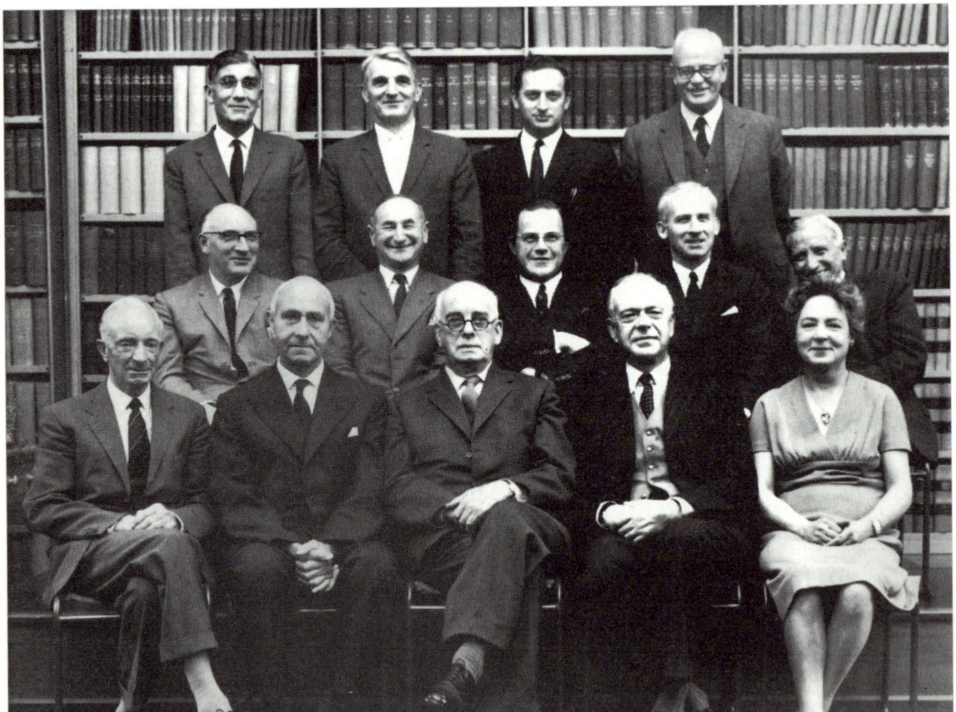

Figure 26 The statutory PHLS Board at its meeting in July 1963 – the last chaired by Sir Landsborough Thomson. *Top, left to right*: E.E. Hughes, A.A. Miles, C.K. Whitaker (Deputy Secretary to the Board), J. Stevenson-Logan. *Centre, left to right*: C.H. Stuart Harris, C.C. Stevens, C. Alwyn Smith, D. Thomson, J.R.M. McGregor. *Front, left to right*: A.H. Clough, G.S. Wilson (Director of the Service), A. Landsborough Thomson (Chairman), D.V.T. Fairrie (Secretary to the Board), Joan Taylor (Staff Assessor).

Madeline Barry, Wilson's secretary and the single whole-time member of the PHLS administrative staff referred to in Wilson's 1944 memorandum to the MRC, had indeed carried a very heavy load during the years prior to the establishment of the statutory board. In addition to her duties as Wilson's secretary and protector, she kept all the records on personnel and organized the locum duties of the junior medical staff, as well as instigating all the administrative activities that were called for in Wilson's visits to laboratories. The PHLS had undoubtedly been something of a cuckoo in the MRC nest, and needed to keep a rather low profile in the office, calling on other MRC staff as little as possible.

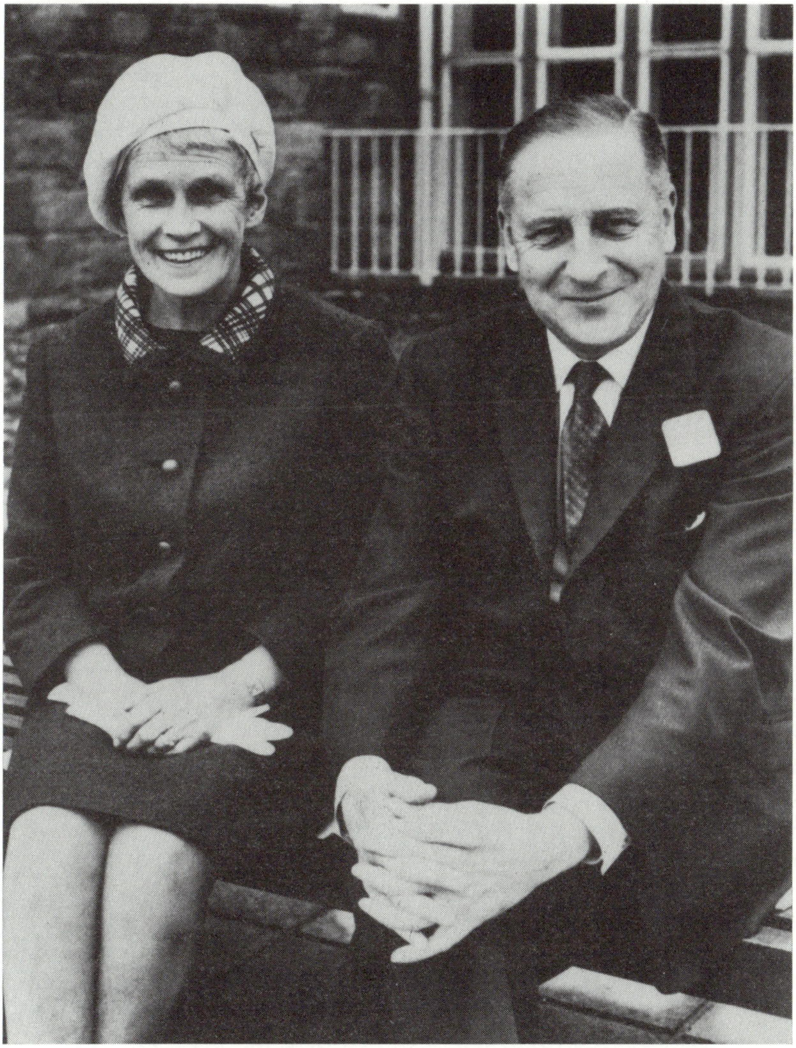

Figure 27 Sir James Howie and Lady Howie, at the Aberdeen meeting of the British Medical Association in 1969.

At the same time as Wilson retired from the directorship of the Service, Sir Landsborough Thomson retired from the chairmanship of the Board, after having been concerned with the Service virtually from its conception, 25 years previously. His contribution was second only to Wilson's in establishing its mode of operation and hence its success. Figure 26 is a photograph of the members of the Board, taken at the last meeting chaired by Sir Landsborough Thomson. (Dr E.T.C. Spooner and Professor A.W. Downie were absent.) Thomson was succeeded as Chairman by Dr E.T.C. Spooner, the Dean of the London School of Hygiene and Tropical Medicine, and a former member of the staff of the EPHLS.

James W. Howie (*b.* 1907, Figure 27), who succeeded Wilson as Director, had been head of the Bacteriology Department of the Rowett Research Institute in Aberdeen until 1951, when he was appointed Professor of Bacteriology in the University of Glasgow, based at the Western Infirmary. In that post he had had the responsibility for providing the clinical bacteriology services for the hospital but, unlike other university bacteriology departments in Scotland, not the public health bacteriological services for the city. Howie had, however, been instrumental in establishing some joint hospital/public health laboratories in the South-West Region of Scotland. While in Glasgow, Howie became especially interested in the problems of sterilization and demonstrated that some of the hospital sterilizers in use were incapable of killing the spores of the tetanus or gas gangrene bacilli. He was instrumental – thanks partly to his mastery of the English language – in alerting pathologists and hospital administrators to the generally unsatisfactory situation. Howie also played a large part in the foundation of the College (later the Royal College) of Pathologists, and was to become its second president.

The Service that Howie joined in 1963 had been through difficult years preceding the establishment of the statutory Board, with the threats of take-over by the Ministry, and there was still uncertainty as to how the future relations between the new Board and the Ministry would develop; indeed there were fears in some quarters that the Service was being deliberately run down by the Ministry by the use of financial pressure. These concerns over the whole future of the Service can only have been accentuated by the reticence that Wilson had always displayed over discussions of future policy. Howie had, therefore, to re-establish confidence as to the future among the staff; but he also soon found that the Service was indeed being inadvertently run down because it had not been receiving the appropriate annual allowance of funds to compensate for inflation. The 1950s seem to have been a period when, for the most part, the financial management of the Service was fairly relaxed and Wilson had been able to leave the problems of finding the necessary funds to Fairrie, and ultimately to Landsborough Thomson, in the MRC office. With the establishment of the statutory Board, the PHLS financing was separated from the Council's and a much firmer and more formal negotiating position had to be established. Howie's aim was to secure adequate funding from the Ministry, while at the same time maintaining freedom from undue "interference" by the Ministry, and continuing to give the laboratory directors the academic freedom and encouragement that they had had from the MRC. Before accepting the post of Director, Howie had received assurance from Sir George Godber, the Ministry's Chief Medical Officer, of full support for the future of the Service and, taking part himself in the negotiations, was soon able to secure a substantial supplement to the PHLS budget. At the same time it was agreed that some rationalization of the Service was needed, with a reduction in the total number of laboratories. The case for additional staff was supported by the workload studies mentioned elsewhere (p. 94), and was soon accepted. Furthermore, in 1965 it was agreed that the PHLS could have access to the Ministry's research funds. These proved very valuable in supporting several important development projects – particularly computer identification of bacteria and the establishment of a mycoplasma laboratory.

The somewhat equivocal position of the PHLS in relation to the National Health Service was emphasized again when, in 1965, the government announced measures to hold back expenditure, from which hospitals but not the PHLS were excluded. The Board protested that the PHLS was an essential part of the National Health Service, but received simply an assurance that there would be a "very close relationship" between the hospital service and the PHLS in respect of capital funding.

Howie did not share Wilson's fear of leakage of confidential information, and in 1964 he secured the appointment as Deputy Director of the Service of S.T. Cowan, who was already administrative director of the Central Public Health Laboratory; this combination was a whole-time job and Cowan resigned from his post as Curator of the National Collection of Type Cultures, though happily continued to write what are almost satirical papers on bacterial taxonomy until his death in 1976. Cowan was succeeded as Deputy Director of the Service in 1967 by J.C. Kelsey. Among his duties, Kelsey took on for Howie some of the routine visiting of the laboratories; he claimed that his best source of information about the problems of a laboratory could sometimes be the director's wife, while he helped with the washing up. (A striking change from the Wilson era; Wilson very rarely even accepted an invitation to dinner.)

The appointment of a deputy director was part of a more general opening up, and indeed enlargement, of the headquarters office. Howie was also much readier than Wilson had been to discuss policy with the staff, and particularly with Fairrie and his successor as Secretary to the Board, J.D. Whittaker. Howie also instituted a programme of small dinner meetings to precede Staff Committee meetings and at which those present could work through the agenda. (Some saw this as the formation of an inner cabinet, and others as liable to curtail discussion by the full Staff Committee.) Undoubtedly the Staff Committee, which continued its pattern of five meetings a year, seemed able by its discussions to contribute far more to policy than it had in the past, but it was not a decision-making body. Howie himself has said that, while giving the appearance of a hierarchy, the reality of the PHLS administration approached more closely to what he called "democratic direction" (Howie, 1970). With the help of his wife, Winifred (Figure 27), Howie initiated the annual reception for senior staff, to which wives and husbands were invited.

The administration of the Service continued along the lines set from the start, operating without the need for numerous committees or any superfluous bureaucracy. During the 1960s most of the administrative staff in the headquarters office were civil servants on secondment from the Ministry. When Fairrie's retirement from the post of Secretary to the Board became imminent in 1965, the Ministry proposed that he should be succeeded by a civil servant; the Board dissented from this view and wished to make its own appointment. After prolonged discussions it was agreed that the Board might appoint J.D. Whittaker, on secondment from the Medical Research Council, a felicitous solution as Whittaker had been much concerned with the development of the Service while Supplies Officer at the MRC and was well known to many of the Staff. He took up his appointment on 1 April 1968.

As has been mentioned earlier, the measurement of the workloads of laboratories is a topic that has been pursued, with very limited success, both within the PHLS and outside, for many years. As part of his policy to establish adequate staffing levels for PHLS laboratories, Howie invited the Staff Committee to set up a working party on measurement of workload, which he chaired, and which reported in March 1964. It recommended that all laboratories should have at least two senior medical members of staff, but that the actual number should relate to the numbers of specimens received: for example, a laboratory having 80,000 specimens per year (virus specimens each counting as 10) would need four medical staff and some 17 technicians. The "Howie formula" provided a valuable general guide, which was actively quoted by laboratories seeing themselves as understaffed, but less fervently by those already over the norm (several persisted in this happy state for many years). Although the formula was neither accepted nor rejected by a study team from the Organization and Methods Unit of the Ministry which reviewed the workload and non-medical staffing of six selected laboratories, it was undoubtedly helpful in Howie's continuing discussions with the Ministry, and indeed contributed usefully to the Royal College of Pathologists' thinking on staffing of pathology laboratories generally.

A further innovation was the constitution of a committee on laboratory buildings, to enable laboratory directors to play a greater part in planning their own laboratories – a principle bringing mixed blessings, as illustrated by the development of "New Colindale" (p. 131).

The functions of the PHLS

As already noted, Howie had early agreed with the Ministry on the need for some rationalization of the laboratory network, but it was not until 1968 that the Board set up its committee on the organization of the service, to consider a 10-year capital programme. The report of the committee, received in January 1969, provided what was the first comprehensive statement of functions that reflected the actual activities of the Service since the *British Medical Bulletin* survey of 1951 or Wilson's Royal Sanitary Institute paper of 1948 (Wilson, 1948*b*).

The function of the PHLS could be summarized as: "to make a continuous study of how microbial diseases are spread, and what advice should be given for their control". The report emphasized that the PHLS should, as part of the routine microbiological service, isolate, identify and record significant pathogens in different parts of the country – Howie's view that the PHLS should be making detailed observations in a number of representative sample areas. The committee felt that there might be a need for some restriction on the requirement that the laboratories should accept any specimen from a medical officer of health or general practitioner, and, while the laboratories' scope in relation to hospital work needed to be defined, it was accepted that the laboratories would normally undertake some or all of the hospital work for their areas. The committee again dismissed the idea that the PHLS should do all the hospital bacteriology for the country, but considered that it must have access to some. It emphasized the importance of laboratories having at least two consultants, and considered that there would be advantages in concentrating resources into fewer, larger, laboratories. The committee was, for fear of creating alarm and despondency, coy about the number or location of the laboratories that might be closed, but offered to provide guidance to the Director of the Service and the Chairman of the Board. At the October 1969 meeting of the Board it was agreed that the number of regional and area laboratories should be reduced to about 50 over a 10-year period, and it was reported that the Ministry had agreed that resources released by closures might be retained by the PHLS for redeployment elsewhere. This last was a remarkable negotiating achievement; in the case of the withdrawal of the PHLS from a joint laboratory it meant that the hospital authority was landed with all the additional expense.

The Central Public Health Laboratory

Colonel H.J. Bensted had retired from the PHLS in 1956 and after what seemed to have been extended private discussions Dr W. Charles Cockburn, the Director of the Epidemiological Research Laboratory, was appointed "Administrative Director" of the Central Public Health Laboratory. The change in title appears to have reflected both the almost obsessional desire of the reference laboratory directors to have total scientific independence, and some possible squeamishness in having an epidemiologist as "Director" of a microbiological establishment. Cockburn held the post until, frustrated, he left to go to the World Health Organization in Geneva in 1961, when he was succeeded by S.T. Cowan, who also retained his post as Curator of the National Collection of Type Cultures until 1964. Cowan retired in 1967 and was succeeded by J.C. Kelsey, the director of the Disinfection Reference Laboratory. From 1967 the Administrative Director was supported by an "Administrator".

Over the years the independence of the individual reference laboratories increased; while they shared support facilities, such as a media preparation department (though most insisted on preparing their own media as well), an animal department and a photographic department, there was little in the way of sharing of other equipment or facilities, and too little scientific intercourse between departments.

The changes of director and title in the individual reference laboratories are shown in Appendix Table 5. Two new laboratories were opened at Colindale: the Disinfection Reference Laboratory and the Mycoplasma Reference Laboratory. The latter was, in the first few years, paid for by a grant from the Ministry's research funds; it was physically (and scientifically) carved out of the Virus Reference Laboratory. The origin of the Disinfection Reference Laboratory lay partly in J.C. Kelsey's experience while in Peterborough of a case of hospital-acquired tetanus, but largely in the growing realization of the unsatisfactory performance of many hospital sterilizers and the widespread ignorance of the proper use of chemical disinfectants. Kelsey was appointed director of the laboratory, which, like the Food Hygiene Laboratory, had education as an important part of its remit.

The Standards Laboratory for Serological Reagents celebrated its 50th anniversary in 1965; the work of the laboratory had expanded very considerably over the previous few years, particularly in the virological field, and the decision was made to cease to provide laboratories outside the PHLS with a range of bacteriological reagents that could be supplied by the Wellcome Foundation. The Standards Laboratory, however, continued to prepare these reagents for the PHLS and to test the material produced by the Wellcome.

The Colindale Routine Diagnostic Laboratory, later renamed the Diagnostic Reference Laboratory, took over most of the routine diagnostic virology from the Virus Reference Laboratory and did a great part of the virological diagnosis for hospitals in the London area.

Other reference laboratories

In 1959 the PHLS took over the Central Tuberculosis Laboratory at Cardiff, which the Welsh Board of Health had inherited from the King Edward VII Welsh National Memorial Association, and renamed it the Tuberculosis Reference Laboratory. Dr J. Marks remained its director and the laboratory continued to occupy its original premises in the Institute of Preventive Medicine.

In 1961 the Malaria Reference Laboratory, which had been transferred from the Ministry to the PHLS in 1946, was transferred from the PHLS to the London School of Hygiene and Tropical Medicine, ostensibly because the legal officers of the Ministry had doubts on the propriety of a malaria laboratory being administered as part of a bacteriological service! (Perhaps these doubts could have been allayed if the word "microbiological" had, as suggested, been used in the Act. The laboratory was to return to the PHLS in 1980.)

In 1964 a Leptospirosis Reference Laboratory was set up by the London School of Hygiene and Dr L.H. Turner was appointed director; he had been the PHLS reference expert on leptospirosis for some years.

The new Colindale

At its July meeting in 1964, the Board had a paper setting out the need to provide a substantial increase in the laboratory accommodation at Colindale, from the current 44,000 ft^2 to around 100,000 ft^2, if the reference laboratories were to continue on one site; this policy the Board reaffirmed. It was clear that sufficient space could not be found on the current, seriously overcrowded site (Figure 28).

This was the start of a saga that has only now – 21 years later in 1985 – reached its climax. The Board agreed to submit the case to the Ministry early in 1965 and in August of that year the Minister of Health, Mr Kenneth Robinson, visited Colindale and agreed that the laboratory had an important role. In 1966 the laboratory was visited by the Permanent Secretary and the Chief Medical Officer, and the Ministry accepted the Board's view that the provision of space was urgent; it promised to seek a suitable site and offered several, in London, for consideration at the Board's May 1966 meeting. At that meeting Howie proposed, instead, that the laboratory should move to

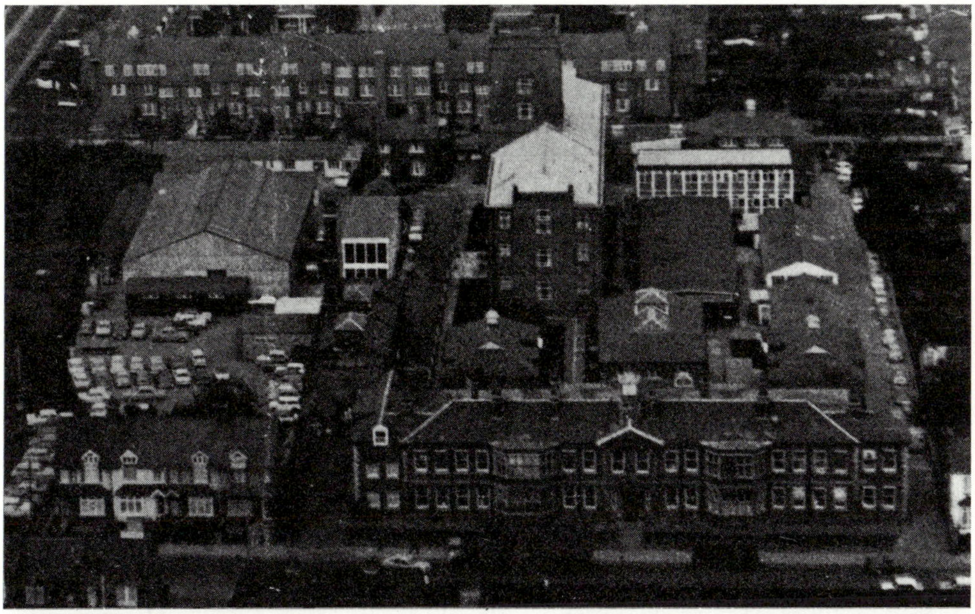

Figure 28 An aerial photograph of the Central Public Health Laboratory, 1972.

Birmingham, where he had been informed that there was an admirable site on the university campus, and where he had been assured of a great welcome by the Vice-Chancellor. Howie was very keen on this proposition, but the Board had serious doubts and set up a committee which visited the site and consulted with the staff. Of the directors of area and regional laboratories, about half would have favoured a move of the CPHL to Birmingham, but of the 11 directors at Colindale, who would have been directly concerned, all but two were against a move and considered that it was preferable to remain at Colindale, even if the space were inadequate. The committee recommended that the CPHL should remain in London, preferably on the adjacent Colindale Hospital site, and did not consider that the upheaval of a move away from London would be justified, even with the advantage of a university site.

In 1968 Robert Matthew, Johnson-Marshall and Partners were appointed architects for the scheme and set about detailed researches into the perceived needs of the directors of each individual laboratory, not, one supposes, realizing that none of them would be in post, even when the building plan came to be finalized. The Ministry finally agreed, in 1969, that the CPHL should be rebuilt in the grounds of Colindale Hospital. By this time, too, the MRC required the space at Park Crescent occupied by the Headquarters Office and it had been agreed that a new set of administrative offices should be provided on the same site at Colindale, despite some contrary advice from the Colindale directors, and the considerable advantages of a site in central London. Thus the headquarters team, which had for its first 15 years been housed in elegant 18th Century buildings overlooking St James's Park (Figure 29, top left), and for its next 12 years in equally elegant buildings overlooking Regent's Park (Figure 29, top right), was

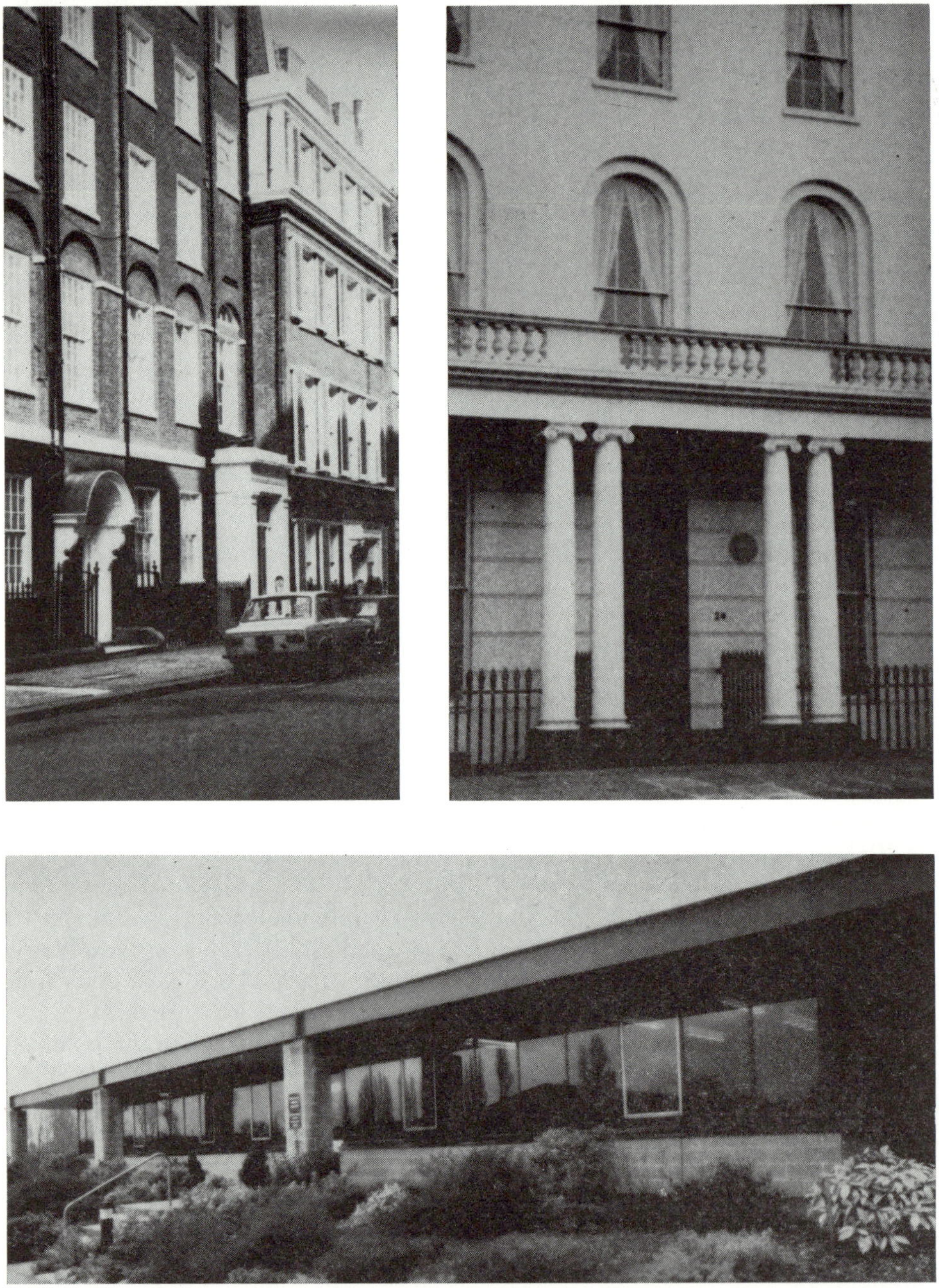

Figure 29 The three headquarters of the PHLS: 26 Old Queen Street (*top left, with the large white doorway*); 24 Park Crescent (*top right*); and 61 Colindale Avenue (*bottom*).

to occupy a lightweight, modern and distinctly idiosyncratic structure overlooking the grounds of an erstwhile tuberculosis hospital (Figure 29, bottom). The elegance of both of the first two offices was paid for by a severe limitation on space (and, in the case of Old Queen Street, a number of floors that were distinctively out of horizontal) and, with the inevitable growth of the headquarters staff attributable to the increased complexity of the administration, the additional space was vital.

Meetings for non-medical staff

Whereas the PHLS laboratory directors met regularly from 1946 onwards, there had been no regular meetings of the non-medical staff. A proposal to rectify this omission with a meeting for head technicians was agreed by the Staff Committee in December 1966 (and estimated to cost £650), though the first meeting – to be part scientific and part social – was not held until 1968. In the meanwhile a meeting of the junior medical and scientific staff was held in 1967. From these beginnings there evolved a tradition of annual scientific meetings, the first, in 1971, for senior technicians (medical laboratory scientific officers; MLSOs), later embracing other non-medical scientific staff, and ultimately emerging as a broadly based scientific meeting open to all grades of staff. Latterly too, the meetings inevitably included sessions for the airing of controversial administrative topics.

Scientific Work of the Service, 1957–69

In the years prior to 1953 almost all the scientific work of the Service had been related in one way or another to the "classical" infections, and the Chief Medical Officer's annual report "On the state of the public health" offered an appropriate text. By 1957–69 the decline in so many of the classical infectious diseases, and the increasing involvement of PHLS laboratories in hospital work, altered the balance. Some indication of this is given by the topics of published work; of 615 items published in 1945–56, some 9 per cent dealt with clinical bacteriology or virology, while of 598 papers published in 1967–9 the percentage was 18. It is not now possible to discover what proportions of the specimens received for examination were derived from hospital patients, but during the period 1957–69 the total number of specimens received rose from 1.8 million to about 3.5 million per annum. The annual number of "sanitary" specimens – food, milk, water and the like – remained fairly constant at about 400,000; a great part of the increase is represented by extra specimens "for the isolation of bacteria" and this certainly largely represents the increase in the general bacteriological work for hospitals. The recognition by Kass (1956) of the value of quantitative bacteriology in the diagnosis of urinary tract infections sparked off a formidable increase in requests for bacteriological examination of urine, which was to result, in the succeeding decade, in this examination constituting about one-fifth of all those requested.

It is not possible to review all the scientific work of the Service here; in the following pages I have referred to the topics that generated most work, or discussion, or seem of particular innovative importance.

Smallpox

Endemic smallpox had left Britain before the start of the period covered by this chapter, but it was still very prevalent in the East and with increasing traffic between Britain and the Indian subcontinent opportunities for importation were considerable. There were a small number of cases each year from 1957 to 1960; in 1961/2 there were five separate importations with a total of 67 cases and 26 deaths. PHLS laboratories were responsible for the distribution of smallpox vaccine and came under great pressure, in consequence of the wide publicity given to the outbreak and the calls for mass vaccination. This vaccination is thought to have resulted in 12 deaths and, coupled with the absence of smallpox in the next few years, led to calls for the abandonment of infant vaccination, finally agreed in 1971.

The Virus Reference Laboratory was the principal centre for smallpox diagnosis, although the university laboratory in Liverpool (Professor A. W. Downie, succeeded in 1965 by K. McCarthy) also offered diagnostic facilities for the North. By 1961 the PHLS laboratories at Leeds and Cardiff were also officially designated for smallpox diagnosis; later Newcastle (1963), Bristol (1967), Portsmouth (1967) and the university department of bacteriology at Birmingham (1967) were added to the list. The Cardiff laboratory was particularly concerned in the 1961 outbreak, examining 243 specimens from suspected patients. The use of gel-diffusion for seeking the antigen in pock contents provided a much faster method of diagnosis than had been available previously. By 1964 the use of the electron microscope had been shown to give very rapid and precise diagnosis ((Nagington, 1964) and was of particular use during the outbreaks of 1966. Unfortunately it was not possible to instal a suitable microscope at Colindale until 1968, although the smallpox diagnostic laboratories all made arrangements to use microscopes in nearby institutions as required. In 1966 there were four outbreaks of variola minor, presumably all arising from a single case now considered most likely to have been the result of a laboratory infection.

Influenza

In June 1957 the Staff Committee was told of the appearance of a new and apparently virulent strain of influenza virus in the Far East, and warned that it could be expected in Britain during the winter of 1957/8. This prediction was amply borne out by the Asian 'flu epidemic that commenced at the end of August. A striking feature of the epidemic was the overwhelming preponderance of staphylococci in the lungs of patients who died of post-influenzal pneumonia, reminiscent of the 1918–19 experience; of 477 fatal cases analysed in a PHLS report (1958*d*), 62 per cent had evidence of staphylococcal infection and the proportion was as high as 88 per cent among the 69 school-age children.

A vaccine made from the epidemic strain of influenza virus was prepared by F. Himmelweit at the Wright Fleming Institute, St Mary's Hospital Medical School, and when used during the autumn of 1958 there was some hint that it might give reasonable protection, a hint that has hardly been supported in the many subsequent vaccine trials in Britain. A number of such trials were conducted, mostly under the auspices of the MRC Committee on Influenza and Respiratory Virus Infections; the PHLS took part in some trials to explore the use of live vaccines (e.g. Andrews *et al.*, 1966) and provided diagnostic back-up for many other trials.

The considerable influenza epidemic of 1967–8 was documented in some detail, thanks to the development of the Royal College of General Practitioners' recording scheme, the availability of figures for new sickness claims, and the large number of PHLS laboratories examining specimens (Miller and Lee, 1969). The laboratories were also able to detect the spread of the next variant – Hong Kong – during 1968, although this strain did not produce its major epidemic until the winter of 1969–70. One objective of the detailed surveillance of the epidemics was the establishment of some measures for prediction, even though, as the Chief Medical Officer wrote in his 1969 report, the advantage to be gained from prediction was "mainly for public reassurance", in the context of persisting memories of the 1918–19 pandemic.

Throughout this period, Hoyle was continuing his investigations into the structure of the influenza virus and the chemical nature of the haemagglutinin and neuraminidase. Hoyle's monograph (Hoyle, 1968) is a masterly summary of the knowledge of the influenza virus accumulated to that date.

Poliomyelitis

In 1957, 4844 cases of poliomyelitis had been notified but the vaccination programme with the killed Salk vaccine was well under way and by mid-1958 some 10 million doses had been issued; notifications declined to 1994 in 1958. The fact that, by 1958, two-thirds of the PHLS laboratories were able to cultivate the poliovirus in HeLa cells made it possible to study the epidemiology of the infection in much more detail. Thus, in 1957–8, 21 laboratories participated in a study of the carrier rate for poliovirus in normal children under five years of age; 124 (1.4 per cent) of 8864 specimens of faeces yielded virus (PHLS, 1958*e*). Eleven laboratories found an average of 27 per cent of the household contacts of patients ill with poliomyelitis to be virus carriers (PHLS, 1958*f*). Spicer, in the Epidemiological Research Laboratory, collaborated in an analysis of all cases of poliomyelitis notified in 1958, which showed that none of them could have been attributable to the polio vaccine (Geffen and Spicer, 1960). This was probably the first adequate vaccine surveillance study to be conducted in Britain and set the pattern for the routine surveillance established in 1962, after the introduction of the live polio vaccine.

Some flagging in the public interest in vaccination, as the incidence of the disease declined, was reversed by the death from poliomyelitis of a well-known footballer and in 1960 the first trials of the live attenuated Sabin vaccine were initiated. Seventeen laboratories participated in a trial involving over 300 infants to determine the optimum dosage schedule (PHLS, 1961*a*) and the clear-cut results provided the Ministry with the information needed so that, in 1962, the Sabin vaccine was generally adopted as an alternative to the Salk. Meanwhile an outbreak of poliomyelitis in Hull in the early autumn of 1961 provided an opportunity to test the effect of the oral administration of attenuated vaccine to a large proportion of the population as a means of aborting the outbreak. PHLS directors from Hull, Newcastle and Leeds played a large part in organizing this programme.

A second large collaborative study, in which 35 laboratories examined faecal samples from 25,000 children to measure the prevalence of enteroviruses, was carried out in 1961 and 1962 (Galbraith, 1966); it revealed a poliovirus carrier rate of 0.86 per cent before the Sabin vaccine programme started, and of 5.27 per cent afterwards. The carrier rates for echoviruses, adenoviruses and Coxackie viruses were also determined.

In 1962 the Epidemiological Research Laboratory took over responsibility for the surveillance of the field safety of the Sabin vaccine and a report in 1965 (Miller and Galbraith, 1965) summarized the experience of 1962–4, concluding that the incidence of vaccine-associated poliomyelitis was no more than one case per million doses given. This surveillance programme, which gave the Ministry confidence in the continued use of live vaccine despite some evidence of vaccine-associated disease in the USA, has continued to the present.

By 1969 the annual poliomyelitis notifications had fallen to 10 and the disease had joined diphtheria in being one for which individual cases generated quite detailed investigations (and often attention by the media) but not one stimulating much original work.

During the latter part of the poliomyelitis epidemic the Chief Medical Officer had several times noted the risk of confusion in the diagnosis of "non-paralytic poliomyelitis" from viruses other than poliovirus, and this was of especial concern in assessing the success of the vaccination programme. In 1953, when the Virus Reference Laboratory first reported its work, the only agents for which diagnostic antibody tests were available were mumps and lymphocytic choriomeningitis; virus cultivation had to be in fertile eggs or animals and was therefore reserved for special cases. This was all changed with the introduction of tissue culture methods from about 1954 and by 1963 an analysis of the reports to the Weekly Summary, not all from PHLS laboratories, recorded the diagnosis among patients with illness of the nervous system of 149 infections with Coxsackie virus, 219 with echovirus, 157 with mumps virus, and only 35 with poliovirus.

Encephalitis

"Encephalitis" has been an entry in the annual reports of the Chief Medical Officer remarkable not only for the stability of the numbers but also for the lack of comment – surprising for a condition responsible for around 100 deaths each year. During the 1960s virological methods were being developed that could be expected to help unravel this problem, though very little seems to have been reported apart from some studies by MacCallum on herpesvirus encephalitis. Incidentally, the Bristol laboratory was the first in Britain to diagnose a case of primary amoebic meningoencephalitis (Apley *et al.*, 1970) – in a child who had played in a muddy puddle – and much later the Bath laboratory caused considerable consternation by finding the organisms in the supposedly healing waters of the Roman Pool.

Echoviruses and other viruses

The late 1950s saw a rapid increase in the number of different viruses that could be diagnosed and a series of papers from the Virus Reference Laboratory documents experience with echoviruses, Sendai virus, adenoviruses, Coe virus and herpesviruses. A very widespread epidemic due to Coxsackie virus B5 was revealed, in 1965, through collaborative studies organized through the PHLS and involving in all 54 laboratories (PHLS, 1967); 1160 infections were detected over the five years 1960–4 and they were characterized by a great variety of symptoms: 280 of 900 patients for whom records were available having had predominantly central nervous system involvement, 200 primarily muscular, 134 respiratory and 77 gastro-intestinal.

After American experience in their Armed Forces, studies were made of the relation of adenoviruses to acute respiratory disease (ARD). In the Royal Air Force, as in the US forces, adenovirus infection was particularly common among recruits and about half the admissions to the sick bay for respiratory tract infection were accounted for by this virus. A series of outbreaks of pharyngo-conjunctival fever in schools were studied by McDonald from the Epidemiological Research Laboratory, Andrews in the Virus Reference Laboratory and their colleagues (Kendall *et al.*, 1957); the characteristic clinical and epidemiological features of the illnesses due to adenoviruses were established. The Chief Medical Officer's report for 1958 had a chapter on "common respiratory diseases" which emphasized the magnitude of their contribution to winter illnesses, and the still distinctly patchy nature of our understanding of their etiology. Among the big gaps were the common cold and epidemic bronchiolitis of infants, considerable outbreaks of which had been reported from various cities.

The MRC Common Cold Research Unit at Salisbury had done quite a lot of work to define the behaviour of the common cold but had not yet isolated a virus. As a follow-up to our own studies of air disinfection with ultra-violet, Lidwell and I set up some quite extensive investigations in the Ministry of Pensions and National Insurance office at Newcastle. We studied the effect of *n*-hexylresorcinol as a disinfectant vaporized into the air, and of an increased ventilation rate, on the reported incidence of colds; neither had any effect. The analysis of the relation of colds to weather was probably of more general interest but all of this work was, as it turned out, somewhat premature in that it antedated by only a short time the recognition of the common cold viruses.

Respiratory syncytial virus was first recognized, in Britiain, by the Bristol laboratory in 1961 and this was soon followed by the finding of it in Birmingham, Blackburn and Manchester: it was clear that one of the gaps identified by the Chief Medical Officer – the etiology of bronchiolitis – was being closed.

Another quite dramatic clarification came in 1962 with Marmion's observation (Goodburn and Marmion, 1962) that the Eaton agent, a supposed virus and the putative cause of atypical pneumonia, was in fact a mycoplasma, shown later to be cultivable – albeit with difficulty – on non-living media.

In conjunction with a Medical Research Council committee, a large survey was conducted in 1962–3 to try to determine the frequency with which cultivable viruses could be identified as the cause of respiratory infections in children (Miller, 1973).

Cytomegalovirus (CMV) infections were studied in Manchester, Bristol and some other laboratories; in Manchester 18 newborn babies, out of 3182 studied, were found to be excreters and 1–4 per cent of women were found to yield CMV from the uterine cervix. Blood transfusion was also shown to be a mode of spread, a route that later became particularly important for patients on immunosuppression after renal transplantation.

Measles

The PHLS Annual Report for 1963 notes that the Epidemiological Research Laboratory was studying the sequelae of measles; a postal inquiry was made in 47 large towns of some 53,000 notified cases. The frequency of serious complications proved to be much higher than expected: in an average epidemic with 35,000 cases, there might be 6000 children admitted to hospital, 600 cases of encephalitis, and 13,000 infections of the middle ear. Deaths were also analysed and although many of the children who died were already suffering from some illness or defect, many were not. These findings certainly swayed the Ministry in favour of mass vaccination against measles, the vaccine for which had been available since 1965 and was already widely used in the United States. The programme, which was started in May 1968, has been carefully monitored by the Epidemiological Research Laboratory to measure the effectiveness of the vaccine protection, especially in the long term, and complications. By 1969 there was good evidence that the programme was proving effective in reducing the incidence of the disease.

Rubella

The Staff Committee seems first to have become interested in rubella in 1965, when it set up a committee which, in 1967, reported that between 80 and 95 per cent of pregnant women had antibodies to the virus. Immunoglobulin was available from the Epidemiological Research Laboratory for the prevention of rubella in pregnant women from 1954 and in 1962 over 20,000 doses were issued. An attempt was made by means of a questionnaire to discover whether it did good. In the absence of a control group this was difficult to determine but the indications were that it did. However, a later study of 5447 pregnant women, in which 652 non-pregnant women exposed to rubella but not given immunoglobulin were also followed, and in which laboratory tests were available to detect infection, gave no evidence for the prevention of infection (PHLS, 1970).

In the late 1960s tests to determine antibody were being developed and these would soon be used to help decide on the management of women who were exposed to rubella during pregnancy (see p. 159) and would also be of value in judging who should receive vaccine, when it became available.

Viral reagents

The great expansion of the virological work of the PHLS from 1956 derived from the introduction of tissue culture for the cultivation of the viruses and the supply of diagnostic reagents. At first HeLa cells were the principal medium used in the area laboratories, but later various other lines became available; in 1959 arrangements were made to supply all laboratories with monkey kidney cells, which were sent out weekly from the MRC Immunological Control Laboratory at Hampstead. At first the diagnostic reagents – antigens for serology and neutralizing antibodies for tissue culture – were prepared in the Virus Reference Laboratory, but after 1954 this work was transferred to the Standards Laboratory for Serological Reagents, which had long experience in the preparation and supply of bacterial diagnostic reagents; by 1963 the Standards Laboratory was sending out virus reagents to 45 PHLS laboratories and around 40 university and other laboratories outside the PHLS. The policy was that new reagents should be studied first in the Virus Reference Laboratory and, when a diagnostic method was ready for general use, the technology would be transferred to the Standards Laboratory, which could develop the method further, prepare bulk reagents or media, and issue them, with guidance as to their use, to the area laboratories. The report by Bradstreet and others (1964) lists the impressive range of materials then distributed. Various commercial sources of reagents for virus diagnosis later became available, and some were adopted as an alternative to in-house manufacture.

Typhoid and paratyphoid fevers

During the years 1958–69 the annual number of cases of typhoid fever generally fluctuated between about 90 and 140, with one year – 1963 – recording 247 due partly to 69 cases from the Zermatt outbreak and to three smaller outbreaks. The figures for paratyphoid fever varied much more, from 89 to 832 (612 of which were part of an outbreak due to untreated milk). Already there were indications that indigenous typhoid was being replaced by imported infection, at that time more from holiday makers in Europe and North Africa than from the Indian subcontinent. The routine phage typing of strains from all cases continued to illumine obscure incidents, as in 1957 when it revealed that a long series of sporadic cases in West Mersea could be attributed to a carrier, presumably first infected in 1885. Phage typing at Colindale played a large part in establishing and elucidating the typhoid outbreak at Zermatt and both the Enteric Reference Laboratory and the Food Hygiene Laboratory gave assistance in the large typhoid outbreak in Aberdeen in 1964. In a later paper Anderson and Hobbs (1973) demonstrated experimentally the survival of *Salmonella typhi* in cans of corned beef, and showed that it had a selective advantage over *Escherichia coli*, which might otherwise have been expected to reveal the contamination by gas formation.

In the Enteric Reference Laboratory, Anderson extended his studies on the biology of the typing phages and demonstrated mutations of the type-determining phages (Anderson, 1959). By 1965 he had turned to the newly discovered phenomenon of the transfer of antibiotic resistance (Anderson, 1965) and studied the spread of *S. typhimurium* type 29, of which some 1700 strains were received in the laboratory between December 1964 and October 1965, almost all of them resistant to one or more antimicrobial drugs. The origin of the epidemic appears to have been trade in young calves by a particularly active dealer and, according to Anderson's account (which has lost nothing in the telling over the years), only ended when the dealer was killed in a motor accident. Anderson and his colleagues recognized that transferable drug resistance in Enterobacteriaceae was attributable to the combined action of two initially independent elements, the resistance determinant – a plasmid – and the transfer factor; the latter was shown to have many of the characteristics of a phage or prophage.

The PHLS was represented on the Swann Committee, which inquired into "The use of antibiotics in animal husbandry and veterinary medicine", by Howie and Anderson, who were doubtless very influential in pressing the committee to recommend the limitation of the use of antibiotics in animal feeds (Report, 1969).

Traveller's diarrhoea

Traveller's diarrhoea is a well established fact of life for those who travel, and it can be of serious import when it affects Army units on exercises or duty in the warmer parts of the world. Studies by Rowe, who combined duties in the Territorial Army Volunteer

Reserve with his work in the Salmonella Reference Laboratory, of an outbreak in Aden in 1965, showed that up to 50 per cent of the cases could have been the result of infection by a single serotype of *Escherichia coli*. The story was shortly to be taken up in more detail as the enterotoxins of *E. coli* became known.

Food poisoning

Food poisoning naturally maintained its position as one of the most important areas of work for the PHLS throughout the period 1957–69 (Figure 21, p. 63). In 1957, 7071 incidents had been recorded, among which 4218 were attributable to salmonellas; in 1968 the 5084 included 3796 due to salmonella, and, while recognition of various new sources of infection often led to methods for their control, changes in feeding habits and in food sources continued to replenish the pool of infection.

Imported feedstuffs and fertilizers were found by Walker in the Maidstone laboratory to be frequently contaminated with salmonellas and a committee set up in 1957 reported a prevalence, for instance, of 48 per cent in bone products, 47 per cent in compound protein meals and 14 per cent in marine products used in feedstuffs (PHLS, 1959*b*). This topic returned frequently to the Staff Committee discussions over the next few years as it was appreciated how the feedstuff contamination was resulting in endemic infections in the food animals, particularly pigs and poultry. The latter were of great importance because of the enormous growth of the broiler industry. This growth was noted in the Chief Medical Officer's report for 1966, when the consumption of table poultry was estimated as 266 million birds per year, as compared with only 25 million 10 years previously. Although the Chief Medical Officer then remarked that food poisoning attributable to poultry meat had been uncommon, this was not to be the picture over the next few years. An outbreak of gastroenteritis due to *Salmonella virchow* in a maternity hospital, in which a total of 40 mothers, babies and staff were ultimately affected, originated from the symptomless mother of the index infant, and she had almost certainly been infected through eating spit-roasted chicken.

The incidence of salmonella infections due to contamination of food animals led to the establishment of a joint committee between the PHLS Staff Committee and the Animal Health Division of the Ministry of Agriculture, Fisheries and Food; this committee has, over the years, provided a very useful forum for presenting to the veterinarians information on human infections derived from animals that are themselves often in no way inconvenienced by the microbes pathogenic for man.

Among the various sources of salmonella infection investigated by PHLS laboratories during the late 1950s and 1960s were flour, following a suggestion that contamination with mouse faeces might lead to a significant hazard in bakehouses; contamination of carcase meat in abattoirs; pet turtles, which proved to be a rich source of miscellaneous salmonellas; and coconuts, imported from unhygienic sources in Ceylon and used in confectionery that often provided a good growth medium. The elimination of the last was a valuable contribution to the prevention of salmonella infections.

Canned foods are, in general, remarkably safe products, but an epidemic of typhoid fever in Yorkshire in 1954, investigated by the district medical officer in collaboration with PHLS laboratories and epidemiologists (Couper *et al.*, 1956) had been convincingly attributed to infection from canned tongue. The cans were known to have been cooled in untreated water drawn from a large river, downstream from a city sewage outfall. It was postulated that typhoid bacilli from the water could have entered the can through a minute defect in the seal. The authors cited four other outbreaks apparently due to canned meat. Subsequently their ideas as to the origin of these outbreaks were substantiated by work on salmonella food poisoning associated with canned meat from Bechuanaland, and, much more dramatically, by the Aberdeen outbreak of typhoid fever in 1964; this was shown to be associated with the use of untreated water from the River Plate for cooling the cans.

Around 1959 PHLS laboratories investigated several outbreaks of staphylococcal food poisoning traced to canned food, in this case peas. Investigations in conjunction with the Food and Vegetable Canning and Quick Freezing Research Association again confirmed that it was possible for material to be sucked into cans during cooling (Bashford *et al.*, 1960).

Food poisoning attributable to *Clostridium welchii* (now *Cl. perfringens*) continued to be a major interest of the Food Hygiene Laboratory (see Hobbs, 1965) and indeed the Chief Medical Officer noted in his 1960 report that this bacterium was responsible for nearly half the "general" outbreaks reported; and again in his 1966 report: most large outbreaks were due to *Cl. welchii.* Many of the outbreaks were in schools and other institutions where stewed meat was prepared in such large quantities that cooling was inevitably slow; but often too little attempt was made to inhibit bacterial growth by refrigeration.

The imminent accession of the United Kingdom to the European Economic Community raised problems, for many European countries had adopted bacteriological standards for foods, and had required medical or bacteriological examination of food handlers, neither of which has had much support in Britain. It is true that a PHLS Committee (PHLS 1949*b*) had advocated some bacteriological standards for ice-cream, but a study that was made of the grading of fresh cream advocated reliance on tests for the effectiveness of the heat treatment, rather than on bacterial counts (PHLS, 1958*g*). An attempt was made to define "advisory" standards for shellfish; when much later similar advisory standards were promulgated for frozen prawns, it became apparent that these were imported in such large containers as to make statistically valid sampling impracticable. The PHLS and the Ministry have consistently maintained that intelligent inspection and monitoring of food-production processes and environments are the best guides to safety. There was considerable discussion, which continued for years, on the possibility that one could assess the general hygienic state of food processes or environments by "general" bacterial counts, and laboratories are often asked by inspectors to examine swabs or other specimens for total bacterial count. The same discussion has gone on in relation to hospital hygiene and with the same conclusion: that environmental sampling is rarely justifiable on critical scientific grounds, but may on occasion be a useful camouflage for inspectors.

The published reports, and the reported Staff Committee discussions on food poisoning, naturally concentrate on the incidents in which a specific microbe can be implicated, but there are many incidents and outbreaks in which no microbe is found. As the tally of microbes recognized as pathogens increases, and as new methods of cultivation become available, the number of outbreaks with source unrecognized should decline: the recognition of *Cl. welchii* in the 1950s is a good example. No "new" pathogens seem to have emerged in the 1960s, but a pointer to the future was Moore's study of "non-bacterial gastroenteritis" in a seaside town; the 1970s were to see several new putative pathogens.

Brucellosis

Brucellosis had always been a topic of interest to the PHLS and work on methods for testing for brucellas in milk has already been mentioned. In 1960 the Chief Medical Officer reported that the Ministry of Agriculture, Fisheries and Food (MAFF), having successfully completed its plans to eradicate bovine tuberculosis, was starting a survey to determine the prevalence of brucella infections in dairy herds; a PHLS report (PHLS, 1961*b*) revealed that of 11,450 milk samples examined in 1959, 4.8 per cent showed evidence of brucella infection. (A previous study using a more sensitive method, carried out in 1955, had found 11.3 per cent of milk samples to be positive.) There were several Staff Committee discussions over the next few years on the difficult problems of serological diagnosis in man as well as on the testing of milk samples. A subcommittee considered that it was necessary to use three serological tests – agglutination, complement fixation, and anti-human globulin – for the most effective diagnosis. Henderson, in the Worcester laboratory, and Robertson at Preston were particularly active and their work highlighted the considerable prevalence of infections – overt or covert – in veterinarians. By 1966 it was considered that probably some 70 per cent of persons with brucellosis were infected by contact with cattle.

The Ministry of Agriculture, Fisheries and Food had started a vaccination programme for dairy herds using the S19 attenuated strain of *B. abortus* in 1961; in 1966 it introduced an eradication scheme and this programme has resulted in a steady decline of brucellosis in man.

Pasteurella *infections*

Dr N.S. Mair, the director of the Leicester laboratory, developed a reference service for *Pasteurella* (now *Yersinia*) infections and was the first to recognize cases of mesenteric adenitis due to *P. pseudotuberculosis* (Mair *et al.*, 1960); he organized a survey in many parts of the country that revealed serological evidence on infection in 102 individuals, 84 of whom had had an operation for "appendicitis".

Toxoplasmosis

Rather similarly, the reference facilities for toxoplasmosis were developed outside Colindale, in this case in the Swansea, Tooting and Leeds laboratories. These laboratories not only provided a diagnostic service for hospitals and PHLS laboratories, but also made studies of improved diagnostic methods.

Leptospirosis

The Leptospirosis Reference Laboratory found the Patoc complement fixation test to be a satisfactory diagnostic method, and was able to make this complement fixation antigen available to PHLS laboratories, so that tests for leptospirosis could readily be included in routine serology.

Hospital-acquired infections

Interest in hospital-acquired infections increased considerably in the second half of the 1950s and, as already noted, the Chief Medical Officer had in his 1956 report commented on the need to discover its real incidence (p. 76). He returned to the topic in 1958, writing that, "Foremost among present-day problems in the field of preventive medicine is the control of pyogenic infection in hospitals". By 1957 a number of area laboratories were being called on to investigate outbreaks of infection, and the Staphylococcal Reference Laboratory was receiving increasing numbers of collections of strains for phage typing. The staphylococcus of phage-type 80/81, originally recognized by Rountree in Australia in 1953, was first detected in Britain in 1954 and by 1957 strains of this type were found in over 40 per cent of the outbreaks investigated by the reference laboratory. The activities of this one memorable strain undoubtedly generated a great deal of interest in hospital infection and in 1957 the Staff Committee set up a subcommittee to devise a survey of the incidence of surgical wound infection. The study, which took place between 1957 and 1959, yielded good clinical and bacteriological records on 3276 surgical wounds and revealed an attack rate for frank sepsis of 9.4 per cent (PHLS, 1960); it was the first broadly based incidence survey to be reported. As important as the general study of incidence was the computer analysis of individual risk factors by Lidwell (1961) – one of the first applications of the new electronic computers in epidemiology.

The Staphylococcal Reference Laboratory collaborated in a long series of studies with Professor R.A. Shooter at St Bartholomew's Hospital, in which we were fortunate enough to be able to introduce some structural modifications to a surgical ward, and to conduct very detailed bacteriological studies of patients, staff and environment. Both at St Bartholomew's Hospital, and in parallel studies by Blowers in Middlesbrough, outbreaks of staphylococcal wound infection due to single carriers among the staff were observed. At St Bartholomew's it seemed that the isolation of patients infected with, or carrying, epidemic strains could prevent spread, but it has to be said that subsequent studies have shown that effective isolation of relevant sources is very difficult.

The 1960 study of surgical wound infection was followed by two further large collaborative studies on the frequency of infection in patients in medical wards (PHLS, 1965*a*) and on the frequency of staphylococcal infection in patients coming to necropsy (PHLS, 1966). The former revealed a frequency of recognized infection of 5.7 per cent on some 7000 patients; the latter showed 10 per cent of about 600 patients dying in hospital to have significant staphylococcal infection.

Another concept arising from these studies was that of the "dangerous disperser", perhaps analogous to the dangerous nasal carriers of haemolytic streptococci revealed by Hamburger's studies in the United States. Studies of dispersal of staphylococci by carriers continued for some years both in the PHLS and elsewhere but although sometimes it seemed that profuse dispersal from a carrier site or lesion could be the origin of an outbreak of infection, there were many examples of dispersal, sometimes giving rise to high concentrations of staphylococci in the air, that did not cause any trouble. Both the capabilities of the staphylococcus and the susceptibility of the people in the environment must be important. Blowers and McCluskey (1965) described experiments with various types of clothing designed to prevent dispersal of bacteria from surgeons' skin.

Interest in the airborne transfer of infection switched from respiratory tract infections to surgical wound infections. Blowers was able to persuade the Newcastle Regional Hospital Board to build him a mock-up operating theatre in which he studied the clearance of airborne clouds of bacteria (Blowers and Crew, 1960), while Lidwell and I visited a number of operating rooms in the London area and used a gas tracer method for defining the pattern of ventilation. The MRC Committee on Hospital Infection incorporated much of this work in what proved to be a somewhat over-elaborate set of recommendations for the design of operating suites (MRC, 1962) which were taken up in a Ministry of Health Building Note and led to the construction of some very complex departments, tending to need more nursing staff than were actually available. Although the detail may have been over-elaborate, the studies of Lidwell, Blowers and others were very important contributions to the developing philosophy of the design and ventilation of operating suites.

A contribution with wide-ranging effects was Moore's (1963) account of the work of a member of the nursing staff specifically appointed to monitor the incidence of infection and to help in the control of its spread; the value of the "infection control nurse" is now well recognized in all developed countries.

The widespread interest in hospital infection naturally led to interest in sterilization and disinfection. The possibility that hospital blankets might be an important vehicle for spread stimulated several studies of possible methods for their disinfection, and was one of the reasons for the constitution of the PHLS Committee on Formaldehyde Disinfection (p. 76) which reported in 1958. A report by the Nuffield Provincial Hospital Trust (1958) on "Present sterilization practices in six hospitals" made grim reading, as had the report from Glasgow by Howie and Timbury (1956). The PHLS did not play a very great part in the development of hospital autoclaves that followed these reports, but was concerned to improve disinfection practices. A Disinfection Reference Laboratory was opened at Colindale in 1960, with J.C. Kelsey as director; its remit was to study and advise on all aspects of disinfection in hospitals and elsewhere. This laboratory produced a wealth of valuable advice, much of which was summarized in the PHLS Monograph *The Use of Chemical Disinfectants in Hospitals*, published in 1972 (and recently revised as *Chemical Disinfection in Hospitals*).

The study of hospital-acquired infection during the 1950s and early 1960s was almost entirely the study of cross-infection with antibiotic-resistant staphylococci. The introduction of penicillinase-resistant penicillins in 1960 and the subsequent – whether consequent cannot be judged – decline of the virulent epidemic staphylococci, led to widespread interest in hospital infection with Gram-negative pathogens, though it seems to have been some years before this became a major topic of interest in the PHLS. The Cross-Infection Reference Laboratory (the successor to the Streptococcus, Staphylococcus and Air Hygiene Laboratory) developed methods for the type-identification of *Pseudomonas aeruginosa* (Wahba, 1965) and a number of laboratories investigated small outbreaks. The development of haemodialysis for patients with renal failure prompted the establishment, in 1967, of a subcommittee to look into the risks of infection; its report, published in 1968, pointed to three areas of concern to microbiologists – the hepatitis risk, shunt sepsis and the hygiene of haemodialysis equipment – and offered guidance on appropriate preventive measures (PHLS, 1968).

The analysis of post-operative clostridial infections, often leading to gas gangrene, by Parker (1969) was important in demonstrating that their origin was more often the patient than the environment; a case of gas gangrene had often led to the closure of operating theatres (and not infrequently requests for the building of new theatres) on the grounds that the infection was extrinsic in origin.

In the Staphylococcal Reference Laboratory, as in the Enteric Reference Laboratory, the routine of typing-phage production and type identification led to more intimate studies of the phages and their hosts. Elizabeth Asheshov with various collaborators showed how the acquisition or loss of type-determining phages by staphylococci could alter their phage type, and how this could explain the change in prevalence from "type 80/81" to "type 52/52A/80/81" in the field (Rountree and Asheshov, 1961). Building on this work, Jevons and Parker (1964) were able to postulate an evolutionary history for a number of strains of antibiotic-resistant staphylococci prevalent in hospitals, while Asheshov studied the behaviour of the genetic elements determining resistance (see, for example, Asheshov, 1969).

Streptococcal infections

The investigation of small outbreaks of infection due to haemolytic streptococci constitute part of the bread and butter work of all area laboratories, but local circumstances have often encouraged some special interest. In the 1950s Payne had studied, and tried to control, outbreaks in residential schools in Yorkshire. In the Cambridge laboratory, Fry and Joan Boissard developed very close links with general practitioners and medical officers of health in East Anglia: they were particularly interested in the control of dangerous, nasal, carriers by means of sulphonamide snuffs. In the Streptococcal Reference Laboratory, Margaret Holmes and I made an extensive study of the prevalent sore throats in a residential orphanage (Holmes and Williams, 1958). Much of this work was stimulated by the recognition that particular serotypes of *Streptococcus pyogenes* are responsible for acute glomerulonephritis. The reference laboratory collaborated with American workers in studies of the epidemiology of nephritis and rheumatic fever associated with streptococcal infection in Trinidad and in Alabama, which demonstrated the importance of skin infections, and the clear difference in serotype distribution between the streptococci from throat and skin infections. This work showed again the great value of using both Lancefield's M and Griffith's T antigens in a typing scheme (Dillon *et al.*, 1967). The extraterritorial activities of the laboratory also included the organization of an international study of the type distribution of *S. pyogenes*.

At the same time Maxted was pursuing more fundamental studies of streptococci: the phages active on Group C streptococci, the protoplasts and L forms of Group A streptococci, and the chemical nature of the surface layers of the cocci. In collaboration with Dutch workers, he was the first to demonstrate that the M type of a clone of streptococci was not immutable (Maxted and Valkenburg, 1969).

Whooping cough

The MRC report of 1956, recording the results of the field trials of vaccines against whooping cough, was followed by encouragement from the Ministry of Health to local authorities to include a pertussis vaccine in their routine childhood schedules. By 1960 the Chief Medical Officer was able to report that all local authorities were indeed offering vaccination, and in 1962 the number of cases notified had fallen to an all-time low of 8357. This reduction was not, however, maintained; preliminary indications that the vaccination programme was not as effective as expected came from the Manchester laboratory's experience in 1963–4 (PHLS, 1965*b*). In 1966 the Staff Committee was alerted to the possibility that there had been a change in the prevalent serotypes of *Bordetella pertussis*, and set up a subcommittee to plan a full study. This study was completed in 1968 (PHLS, 1969) and showed that at least some of the vaccines in use before and during 1967 were apparently not inducing satisfactory protection. Manufacturers had subsequently increased the antigen content of the vaccine, but it was not yet possible to judge the outcome of this change. An indication of troubles to come was a brief report of some adverse reactions to the vaccine from the Portsmouth laboratory.

Tuberculosis

In the 1950s the PHLS's interest in tuberculosis was concentrated on studies of improved laboratory diagnostic methods and on the emerging appreciation of the hazards for laboratory workers. These interests were continued in the 1960s with special concern for the hazards associated with the methods used for determining drug susceptibility – often utilizing fluid cultures (Marks, 1961). Several laboratories collaborated in a study of the excretion of tubercle bacilli by guinea-pigs infected in diagnostic tests; it was held – in 1962 – that it was essential to use animal inoculation in seeking tubercle bacilli in urine and some other critical specimens.

The prevalence of drug-resistant strains was studied by a PHLS committee (PHLS, 1961*c*), and a central register of such strains was established in the Tuberculosis Reference Laboratory in 1962, where Marks (1961) had developed the important concept of "modal resistance". In a report in 1965, Marks demonstrated the very great discrepancies between the results of susceptibility tests in the reference laboratory, as compared with those obtained in the laboratory in which the strain was isolated and first tested. The technical difficulties of achieving reproducibility in drug susceptibility tests, as well as the risks of infection, led to the proposal to concentrate as much as possible of this work in eight "regional centres for tuberculosis bacteriology", which were approved in 1967, and which have over the years carried out most of the tests for PHLS laboratories and a great number of those for hospital laboratories.

Marks, in Cardiff, and Collins, in London, studied the classification of the so-called "anonymous", "atypical" or "tuberculoid" mycobacteria, and published classifications and studies of their prevalence and importance (see Marks, 1969).

The Third Phase: 1970–80

The evolution of the PHLS during the 1970s consisted very largely of consolidation of the developments initiated previously. Towards the end of the period, however, there was a major expansion in the field of epidemiology, and the start of a new era with the inclusion of the Centre for Applied Microbiology and Research at Porton Down within the responsibilities of the PHLS Board. No account of the work of that Centre is included in the present essay (see pp. 163–164).

Administration of the PHLS

The 1970s were to see a considerable increase in the activity of the Board and a substantial growth in the central administrative office of the PHLS. Dr Spooner was succeeded as Chairman of the Board in 1972 by Dr C.E. Gordon Smith, like Spooner before him Dean of the London School of Hygiene and Tropical Medicine and a former director of the Microbiological Research Establishment at Porton Down. I accepted the invitation to succeed Howie as Director of the Service from 1 October 1973; since leaving the PHLS in 1960 I had held the chair of bacteriology at St Mary's Hospital Medical School, where I had also latterly served as dean.

In 1975 J.E.M. Whitehead, who had directed the Coventry laboratory since 1958, joined the headquarters office as a second deputy director of the Service; he succeeded J.C. Kelsey as Deputy Director in 1976, when Joan R. Davies, the director of the Guildford laboratory, was appointed a part-time deputy director of the Service, with special responsibility for food and environmental bacteriology.

In 1977 J.D. Whittaker retired from the post of Secretary to the Board; the arguments of 1967–8 were repeated, with the DHSS wishing to see a civil servant seconded to, or at least offered, the post, and the Board wishing to advertise and employ its own senior officers. The Board's view prevailed, and R.S. Sawyer, previously district general administrator in the Clywd Area Health Authority, was appointed. Over the next few years there were many changes in the senior administrative officers, and the policy was accepted that they should be the direct employees of the Board rather than civil servants, seconded from the DHSS. The advantages of this policy have certainly included the possibility to draw from a wide field of experience, but the disadvantages, always stressed by the Department, of limited career prospects must certainly have contributed to the rather rapid turnover of staff.

In 1969 the Board had initiated the policy of having one of its four meetings each year in one of the laboratories outside London; these meetings were residential, and arranged so that members could have informal policy discussions in addition to the formal Board meeting. At most other meetings of the Board a director of one of the laboratories gave an account of the work of his unit. As a further means of informing the Board of the activities of the reference laboratories, a series of scientific review committees were constituted, each with the remit to examine the work of one laboratory and to offer guidance on its future policy; the first was convened in 1979.

The Board thus became more familiar with the work and the staff of the Service than it had been, but the tradition persisted that the Director and Secretary were allowed to get on with running the Service without having repeatedly to seek authority from the Board. The climate of opinion in the 1970s, coupled with the recent experience that both I and Sawyer had had of National Health Service administration, meant that we had to have formal and informal consultation with the staff on far more of the policy matters than in the past. The Staff Committee continued to debate and advise on all manner of topics; from 1977 its meetings were renamed "Directors' Meetings" and reduced to four a year, while other meetings were arranged for discussion of particular topics at which both directors and other senior medical and non-medical staff could attend.

I had an easier job than Howie in taking on the directorship, as the Service had been progressing steadily in the previous few years. I believed that if medical microbiology was not to be relegated to the status of a poor relation in the hospital laboratory services, it had to shake off a "string and sealing wax" philosophy and that the Service ought to be active in employing the emerging opportunities for mechanization, automation and other new diagnostic techniques. We saw the provision of an adequate number of electron microscopes as the appropriate way in which funds available following laboratory withdrawals could be used. The development of automated equipment has proved a much slower process than I had hoped, but by the end of the 1970s there were a quite impressive number of instruments in use, and the application of computers to routine work was beginning to be practical (Figure 30).

The functions of the PHLS

By 1970 the situation had been reached that almost all the PHLS laboratories were in effect hospital microbiology laboratories differing from the other 300 or so NHS microbiology laboratories in their direct scientific and administrative links into the PHLS Board and the Director of the Service, and in their explicit commitment to the support of the community health services under the direction of the local medical officer for environmental health and the chief environmental health officer. At the same time, they had clear and formal responsibilities to the hospital administration for the provision of clinical microbiology services.

The competing claims of the acute clinical microbiology for the hospitals in which the laboratories were situated, and the public health microbiology and epidemiology for the wide community, were still recurrent topics of debate, both in the Staff Committee and in the Board. At the July 1974 meeting of the Board, which was held in Liverpool, there was general support for the conclusions of a Board subcommittee that involvement in hospital work was an essential part of the PHLS's functions, and that

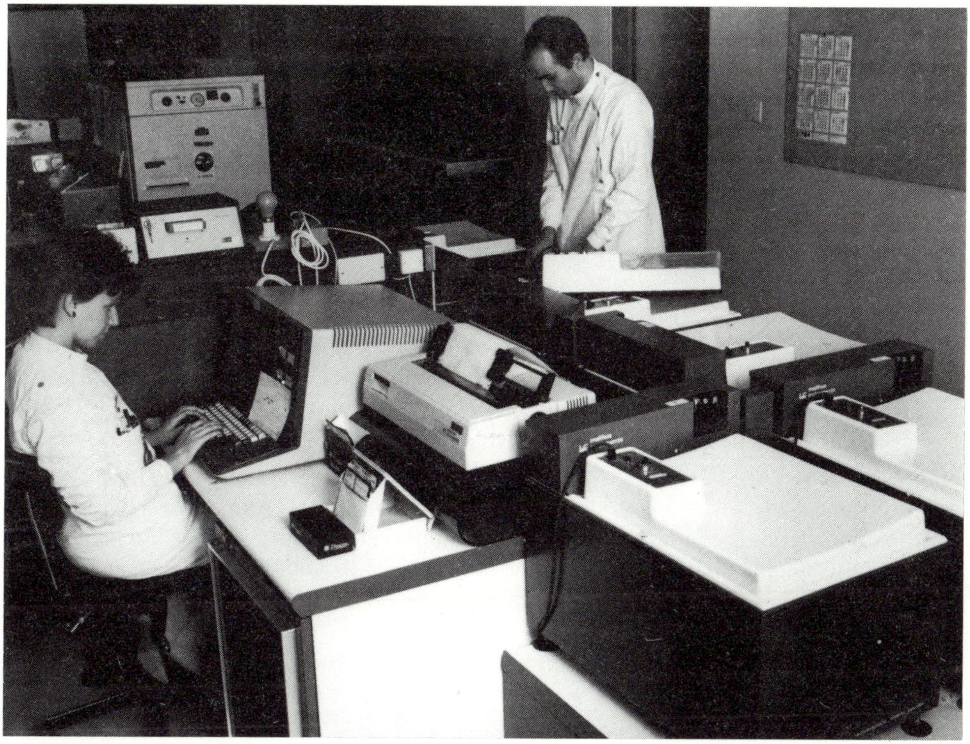

Figure 30 Malthus equipment for automated blood culture developed at the Cambridge Public Health Laboratory.

this implied that all laboratories should have at least two consultants if both hospital and public health work were to be properly covered. Expansion of the epidemiological cadre was also to be encouraged. Next year, at the 1975 summer meeting in Portsmouth, Brendan Moore, since 1945 the director of the Exeter laboratory, suggested that the PHLS ought to be more strongly oriented to public health work, to be part of a complex network of laboratories and field workers concerned in interdisciplinary surveillance of all aspects of environmental health. He suggested that the PHLS should hive off those aspects of clinical microbiology that have no epidemiological significance (though he did not reveal how these were to be distinguished) and he emphasized the importance of spending more effort on tracing the spread of pathogenic microbes. The idea that the PHLS should be more involved in the non-microbiological aspects of environmental health was raised again in 1976 by Spence Galbraith, at the time of his appointment as director of the new Communicable Disease Surveillance Centre, but the reaction then, as in the previous discussions, was that the PHLS should stick to the last it had been built to fit, while being ready to co-operate to the full with any other agencies concerned with environmental health. Unfortunately, such agencies are lacking, and there remains a real gap in the provision of co-ordinated laboratory and epidemiological services for large areas of public health.

Cost-sharing with hospital authorities

The financial bargain that Howie had struck with the Ministry in 1969, which allowed the PHLS to retain resources liberated by withdrawal from laboratories, provided an invaluable cushion during the acute inflationary period of the 1970s, but there was increasing pressure on the PHLS to arrange equitable cost-sharing bargains with hospital authorities. The way to achieve such equity was far from clear. On the one hand, it was often very difficult to discover just what the *total* cost of any particular laboratory amounted to. In addition to the inherent difficulties of such costing, individual laboratories had developed a great variety of often rather peculiar barter arrangements following the earlier agreement (p. 32), and varying proportions of the staff costs were borne by the hospital or PHLS respectively. But more importantly, it was by no means clear what proportion of the workload should be charged to the PHLS if the Service existed, as Howie had insisted, to monitor the infective diseases of the country. It had to have direct access to the clinical microbiology of the hospitals, where many of the patients with infections of concern at the present were to be found. It was no longer possible to equate "public health interest" simply to specimens sent by medical officers of health or general practitioners. Eventually the Board agreed that, in principle, the costs of joint laboratories ought to be borne equally by the PHLS and the hospital authority. An analysis produced for the Board in 1980 revealed that the proportion borne by the PHLS appeared to vary from about 4 per cent to about 75 per cent of the costs in different laboratories. A start was made in 1980 to review the individual cost-sharing arrangements and to negotiate on a 50 : 50 basis, but one could predict both that a long period would be needed to achieve the desired end, and that a whole variety of reasons would insist that 50 : 50 was not appropriate in particular cases.

Finance, and relations with the Department of Health and Social Security

For most of this period, the PHLS was treated, financially, along broadly the same lines as the regional hospital boards, that is to say that the PHLS Board submitted each year its estimate of the financial needs for the succeeding year, having generally been given an indication of what "growth factor" was allowable; the DHSS eventually responded with a figure for the revenue and capital allocation. During the years of rampant inflation from the mid-1970s various methods were adopted to allow for increases in costs, some reasonably generous, some severely restrictive. The programme of withdrawal from laboratories agreed in 1973 provided some welcome financial assistance. As the trend towards joint laboratories with hospital authorities developed, a mechanism was devised that allowed the PHLS effectively to retain, rather than return to the Treasury, the hospital authorities' contributions to revenue costs, and so to allow the gradual disappearance of the barter arrangements that have been referred to earlier. Although in several years financial crises loomed, it was generally true that the PHLS was provided with sufficient funds to maintain the services, and to allow modest expansion in a few directions. The total revenue and capital expenditure of the PHLS

Board from 1961 to 1980, abstracted from the statutory accounts, are shown in Appendix Table 6.

During the 1970s the relations with the Department of Health's officers proceeded in a fairly low key. The Board's Secretary and Finance Officer were in a position to discuss with the Department's officers the tenor of their respective communications to one another, often before they were committed to paper. On the medical side, there were regular meetings to review the epidemiological situation, attended by the Director or Deputy Director of the PHLS, the director of the Epidemiological Research Laboratory, or later of the Communicable Diseases Surveillance Centre, with the Senior Principal Medical Officer in the DHSS Communicable Diseases Division, and other officers of the health and some other departments. These were, of course, supplemented by numerous other informal meetings, but communicable diseases were by now, except for crises such as the importation of a case of Lassa fever, fairly low in the Department's list of priorities, and no longer occasioned regular meetings of the PHLS Director with the Chief Medical Officer.

Relations with non-medical staff

It has always been a cardinal element in EPHLS and PHLS policy that the constituent laboratories ought to be directed by medically qualified microbiologists. This was undoubtedly because the laboratories were expected to participate in epidemiological investigations in the field in collaboration with, and often on behalf of, the medical officers of health. Moreover, as the clinical microbiological activities of the laboratories expanded, it was important that the director could be seen as a full clinical colleague by the rest of the hospital staff. During the period of this review, only one of the area or regional laboratories had a non-medical director (R.L. Vollum, 1949–65 at Oxford) and only the Food Hygiene Laboratory (throughout its life), the Leptospira Reference Laboratory (from 1978) and the Mycological Reference Laboratory (from 1972), among the reference laboratories, had non-medical heads.

It has also always been the firm policy that the director should carry the total management responsibility for running his or her laboratory, a principle that no one would have felt any need to state until recently. Over the years individual directors have exercised this responsibility in a variety of ways, some distinctly idiosyncratic: one is said to have started the laboratory day with morning prayers, one issued written "orders of the day". But in general the relations between director and staff have been on a straightforward basis of colleagues working within their respective spheres of influence, with the head technicians (later head medical laboratory scientific officers, head MLSOs) having delegated management authority, and often themselves contributing very substantially to the scientific work of the laboratories. Examples that come to mind are N.W. Emberley's work with Jameson on the Teepol medium for water bacteriology, G.H. Sandy's invention of the dip-spoon method for urine bacteriology (Figure 31), G.H. Lowe's long series of studies on trichomonads and J.R. McDonald's contributions to the developments in virology, but there are certainly numerous other examples that could be quoted.

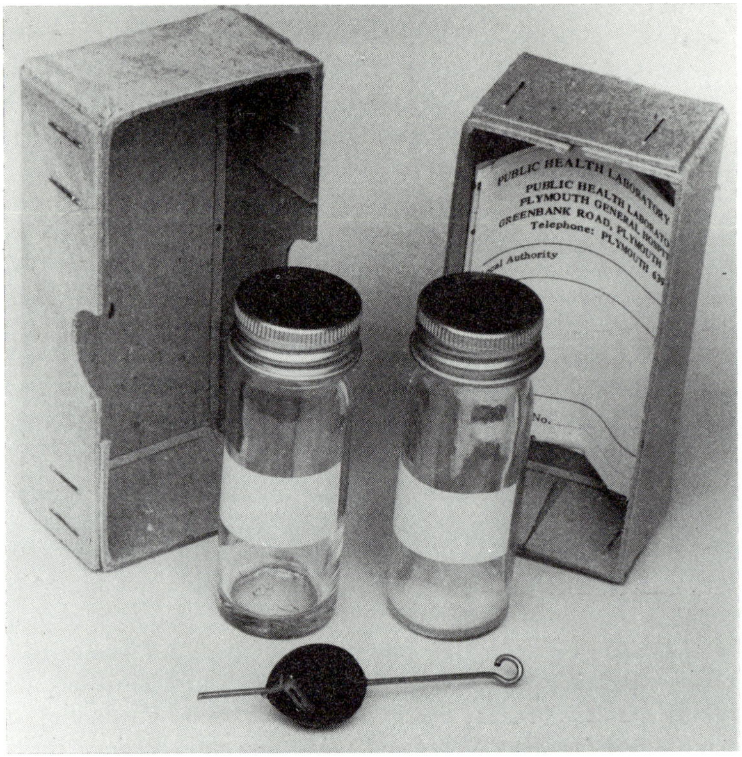

Figure 31 Dip inoculum kit for urine bacteriology developed by G.H. Sandys.

From the early days, non-medical scientific staff were employed in the reference laboratories but very few worked in other laboratories, and at a Board meeting in 1951, when the position of scientists was discussed, it was emphasized that there were few opportunities for them to reach senior posts. By the 1970s the number of scientists had increased substantially and several attempts were made, without much success, to find an acceptable formula that could set out the relative ambitions and responsibilities of the scientists, the MLSOs, and the medical staff. This was at a time when the Institute of Medical Laboratory Sciences had developed a more assertive pose, and was not only suggesting that the traditional responsibility of the director for managing the laboratory budget should be transferred to the head MLSO, but was also anxious to bring the scientists into the Institute's sphere of influence, and to get agreement on a single spine salary. The Board formally endorsed its policy of having the director responsible to it, through the Director of the Service, for the management of the laboratory. In 1976 the Board and the Staff Committee, without I suspect very detailed consideration or consultation, supported the idea of a single-spine salary structure for non-medical staff, but this probably went unnoticed.

At one of the first meetings of the statutory Board, the possibility was raised that the Board might be brought formally within the structure of the Whitley Councils, which

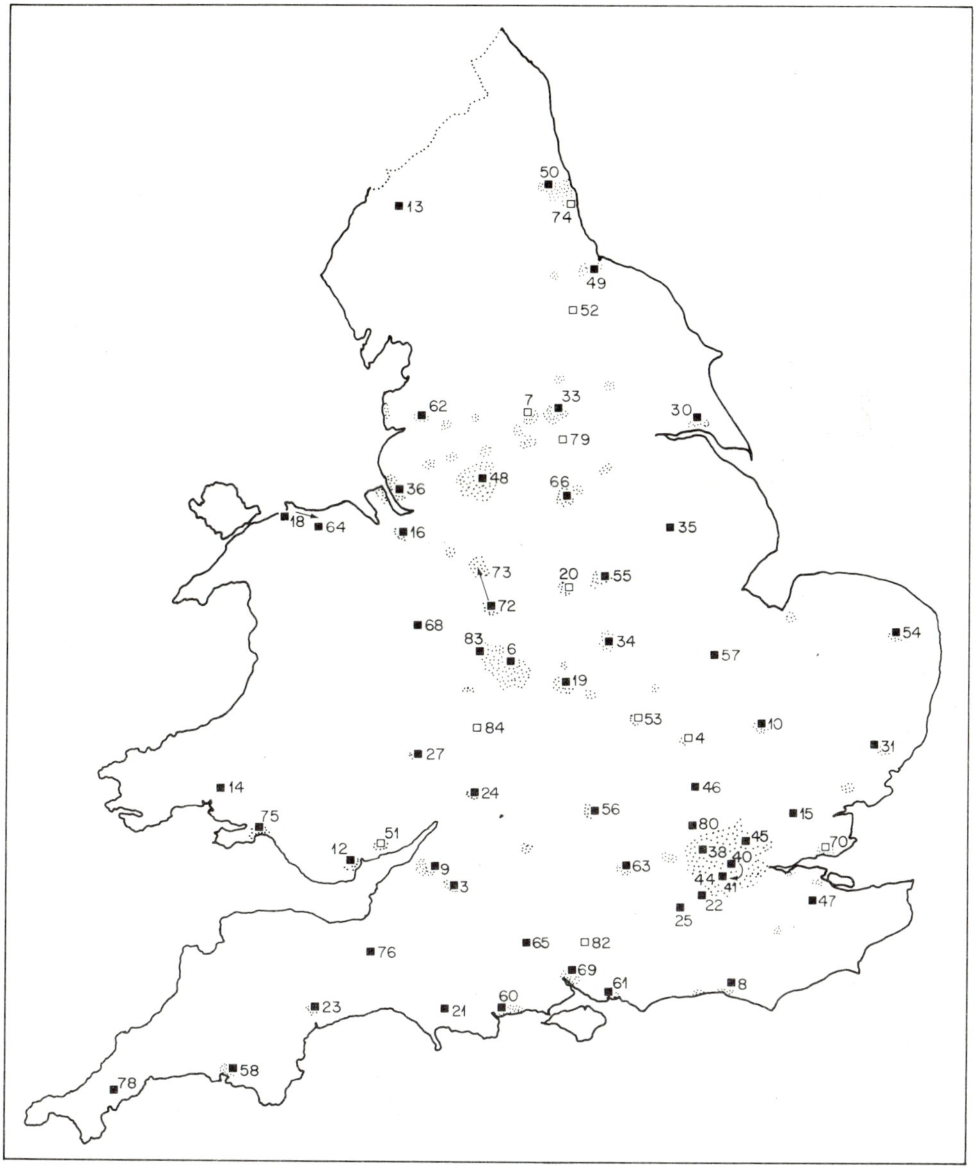

Figure 32 PHLS laboratories, 1970–80. ■, laboratories still operating in 1980; □, laboratories closed between 1970 and 1980. *Note*: Stafford (72) moved to Stoke-on-Trent and London County Hall (40) moved to Dulwich. Numbers refer to names of laboratories as listed in Appendix Table 1.

are the national negotiating bodies for salaries and conditions of service within the National Health Service. The Board had been instructed to bring PHLS terms and conditions into line with those in the National Health Service and it had to seek approval of the Ministry for its salary scales; with a few special exceptions these had always been the same as the National Health Service scales. But this arrangement gave scope for argument: some PHLS staff thought that the Board should try to get special scales to suit what they saw as special circumstances, arising for the different work of public health laboratories. The trade union representing some of the technical staff (and a small number of the scientists) probably also saw this as an opportunity to try to get better salaries or conditions within a relatively small body, such as the PHLS, which could then be cited as a precedent within the larger National Health Service. In the case of the animal house technicians at Colindale, this argument got to the brink of industrial action. In this instance, the PHLS officers were sympathetic to the animal technicians' claims, and eventually an acceptable formula was extracted from the DHSS. But when the Association of Scientific, Technical and Managerial Staffs (ASTMS) demanded the right to negotiate salaries with the Board for all non-medical staff, and when they went further and demanded to be recognized as the sole union representing the non-medical staff, the Board opposed them adamantly. This argument was resolved only after the Arbitration and Conciliation Advisory Service (ACAS) had been brought in to ascertain the views of the staff concerned. The majority view was that they did not want ASTMS to be the one recognized union. Indeed a great many of the staff did not want to belong to any union.

All these arguments seemed to make it certain that the Board should be brought formally into the Whitley machinery. The Board's application was delayed pending the outcome of the ACAS review, and was then held up by union objections in the Whitley Council, but was finally accepted (with some slight reservations) in 1981.

The laboratory network

The Committee set up by the Board in 1968, in the light of the need to increase the staffing of the laboratories without any overall increase in budget, and some DHSS pressure to reduce the number of laboratories, had reported in 1969 with its 10-year

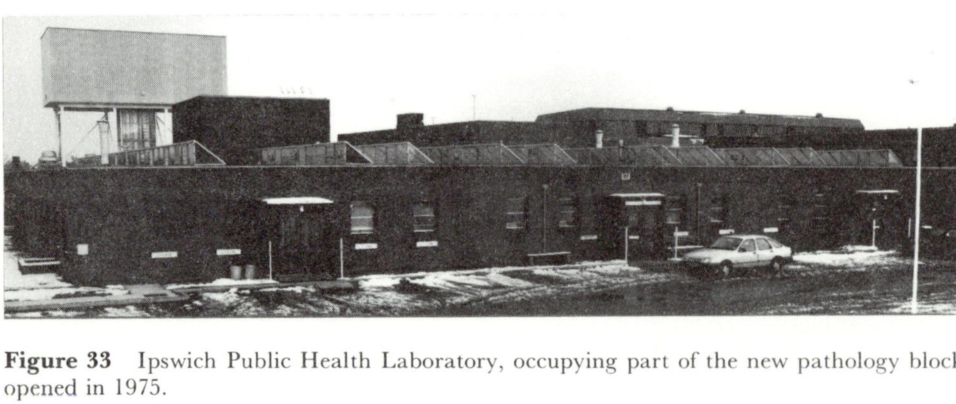

Figure 33 Ipswich Public Health Laboratory, occupying part of the new pathology block, opened in 1975.

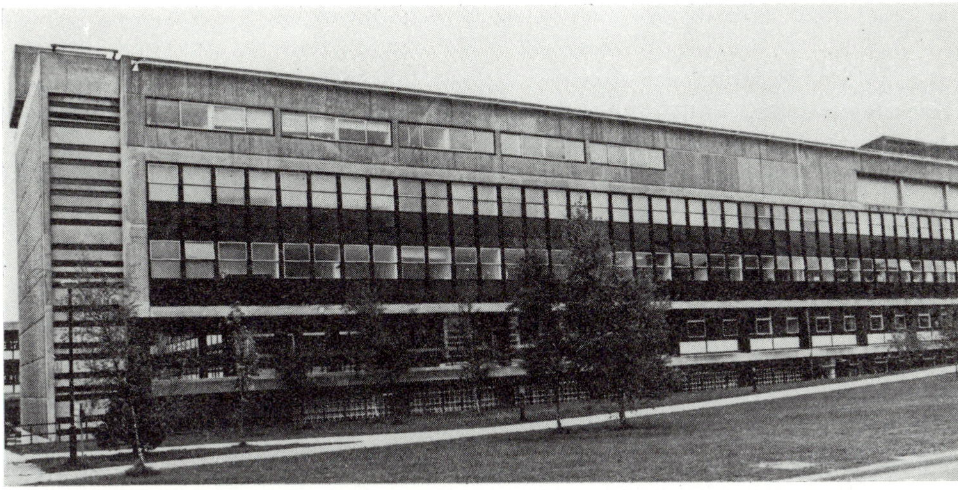

Figure 34 Cardiff Public Health Laboratory occupies part of the new pathology block in the University Hospital of Wales.

plan. What would, in 1980s parlance, be called a "hit-list" of 10 laboratories to be closed or handed over to regional health authorities within 10 years was agreed by the Board in 1970. It was thought that the resources released by these closures should be directed towards strengthening the regional laboratories. In fact, between 1970 and 1980, the PHLS withdrew from 11 laboratories (Figure 32). Two of them, Wakefield and Bradford, were doing only sanitary bacteriology and general practitioner work, but withdrawal from them increased still further the discrepancy between the number of laboratories in the north and the south, as had the 1971 withdrawal from Northallerton. In fact there was a considerable degree of opportunism in the choice of laboratories from which to withdraw and certainly, if a master plan relating laboratory sites to population had been the basis, the Service would not have withdrawn from both Bedford and Northampton. But Hoyle (Northampton) had died in 1952 and Lane (Bedford) had already reached the retirement age. The Derby, Southend and Newport laboratories were close to other PHLS laboratories, and were reasonably regarded as redundant. All the laboratories, other than Wakefield, Bradford and Northampton, had been doing general hospital work, and National Health Service authorities had to accept financial and management responsibility; this must have led to increased costs for the National Health Service, since the PHLS contribution to running costs had generally been substantially in excess of the costs incurred for the public health work. In several cases the PHLS continued to fund one or two posts for a time.

During the 1970s several laboratories moved to locations within general hospitals, usually incorporated in a block with other pathology departments (Figure 33), or within university hospitals (Figure 34). The negotiations often involved Howie and the headquarters staff in extensive consultations (assisted in one case, it is rumoured, by the fact that the vice-chancellor was seeking some help with his golfing technique).

The resources released by the closures were not separately identified and it cannot be said that they were in fact used to strengthen the regional laboratories. Several discussions were held over the years on the distinct functions – if any – of the regional laboratories, but little came of them, largely for the reasons mentioned earlier (p. 42). These laboratories continued to have a larger staff and a greater range of specialist activities than most of the area laboratories, but any move towards developing a hierarchical structure was vigorously opposed. However, in 1976, in response to the recognition of the risks of importation of patients with viral haemorrhagic fevers, it was agreed to establish "special pathogen laboratories" in four of the regional laboratories, and when the plan for enlarging the cadre of epidemiologists was agreed, the "regional epidemiologists" were to be based on regional laboratories, and indeed two were appointed – at Oxford and Manchester.

The reference services

As mentioned previously, the reference services have tended to develop according to the particular ideas of their respective directors, rather than according to a general plan. This has applied both to their scientific activities and to the policy for devolution of work from the central reference laboratory to the area laboratories; there have been both centrifugal and centripetal developments.

Staphylococcal phage typing was an early candidate for devolution; the hospital epidemics of the 1950s made great demands on the reference laboratory and it was thought that local epidemiological investigations would be best supported if the typing could be done reasonably locally, although with reagents supplied from the reference laboratory at Colindale. The peripheral laboratories that took up phage typing were those where the director or some other members of the staff had a personal interest in it. In consequence the devolved typing services were never very rationally distributed over the country, nor did they have defined "catchment areas"; their customers tended to be their friends or former colleagues, who might be far distant. The devolved streptococcal typing laboratories were more rationally disposed and had, on paper, defined catchment areas, but again personal friendships rather than geography often determined which laboratory was used.

Originally all the salmonella serotyping was provided by the Salmonella Reference Laboratory, but in the early 1950s regional centres were established in the Birmingham, Northallerton and Poole laboratories, with the reference laboratory acting for South-East England, and as the parent laboratory for the other three. However, in 1971 it was decided that all reference typing should again be centralized in the Salmonella Reference Laboratory, although area laboratories continued to identify many of the strains they isolated, using the somewhat restricted range of typing sera available from the Standards Laboratory. It was expected that this centralization would facilitate the gathering of a complete national picture, and accommodate more readily the increasing demands for salmonella identification, and even justify the use of mechanical methods (which it did – Shipp and Rowe, 1980).

The phage typing of all salmonellas, including *S. typhi*, was carried out only in the Enteric Reference Laboratory, which had developed the scheme for *S. typhi*, *S. typhimurium*, and some other species, and which received strains not only from the

Salmonella Reference Laboratory and other PHLS laboratories, but also from the Central Veterinary Laboratory, and indeed from many other sources in Britain and overseas.

These centralized arrangements certainly meant that fairly precise information was available on the less common types of salmonellas, but because area and some hospital laboratories were able to identify many of the commoner types, and did not necessarily forward them all to the reference laboratory, the overall picture was less clear.

Devolution of virus diagnostic work was the direct result of Tomlinson's demonstration that HeLa cell cultures for poliovirus could be carried out in routine bacteriological laboratories. There were, on several occasions, suggestions that this devolution had gone too far and, in small laboratories, represented an uneconomic use of resources. But the work was very popular with staff concerned and it is almost certainly the case that much less would have been done, and so our information on the distribution of many viruses would be much less, if all material for virus diagnosis had to be sent to, for example, regional laboratories. In 1971, 13 laboratories were designated as reference laboratories for hepatitis B antibody tests; as the methods became known a number of other laboratories also undertook this work.

The devolution of work on mycology resulted from a definite policy decision by D.W.R. Mackenzie, the director of the Mycological Reference Laboratory; he organized training courses, the supply of reagents, and an information exchange.

Reference services in areas laboratories were not confined to those devolved from the central reference laboratories. In many cases the directors or other members of the staff had developed special interests and expertise; they were recognized as "reference experts", and listed in the PHLS directory so that their advice was generally available. Some individuals outside the PHLS were also designated as "reference experts". Table 3, abstracted from the PHLS Annual Report from 1979–80, indicates the range of reference activities in the area laboratories. These arrangements have generally worked well, provided that the amount of reference work was not too great, although it has sometimes been difficult to find ways of maintaining the somewhat personal reference services on the retirement of the expert, because his successor as director of the laboratory cannot always be expected to continue with the same specialist interest. If the work has to be transferred to another laboratory, there may also be problems when ancillary staff have been provided for the reference work.

Within the Central Public Health Laboratory, there were several changes during the 1970s (see Appendix Table 5). After the death of Dr Patricia Carpenter in 1971, work on shigella species other than *Sh. sonnei* was transferred to the Salmonella Reference Laboratory, thereafter the "Salmonella and Shigella Reference Laboratory". (It never included *Escherichia* in its title though it had been providing a reference service for these bacteria for many years.) Reference work for *Sh. sonnei* was allocated to Dr Joan R. Davies in the Guildford laboratory. In 1978, after the retirement of E.S. Anderson, the Division of Enteric Pathogens was constituted, with B. Rowe as director, to be responsible for all reference work on salmonellas, shigellas (other than *Sh. sonnei*), *E. coli* and some other related enteric pathogens.

The Mycoplasma Reference Laboratory initially had space in the Virus Reference Laboratory but later moved to its own accommodation in the CPHL. The pressure on

Table 3 Reference services in regional and area laboratories, 1981

Laboratory	Diagnostic facilities for virology			Other reference services
	EM	Culture	HBsAg	
Bath	+	+	+	
Birmingham, R	+	+	+	Mycobacteria
Brighton	+	+	+	
Bristol, R	+	+	+	Chlamydia, syphilis serology, gonococcal plasmid typing
Cambridge, R	+	+	+	Legionella, Group A streptococci
Carlisle			+	Fungal serology
Chelmsford	+	+	+	
Chester	+	+		
Coventry	+	+		Klebsiella typing
Dorchester	+	+	+	
Epsom	+	+	+	Coxsackie A viruses
Exeter	+	+	+	
Gloucester		+		
Guildford	+	+	+	*Shigella sonnei*: fungal chemotherapy
Hereford	+	+		
Ipswich			+	
Leeds	+	+	+	Food microbiology, toxoplasma, tubercle bacilli, Group A streptococci, category A virus laboratory
Leicester	+	+	+	Yersinia
Liverpool, R	+	+	+	Mycobacteria, VD serology
London:				
Central Middlesex	+	+	+	
Dulwich	+	+	+	Mycobacteria
Tooting			+	Toxoplasma
Whipps Cross		+	+	
Luton		+	+	Anaerobic bacteria
Maidstone			+	Cholera and other vibrios
Manchester, R	+	+	+	Meningococci, mycobacteria, campylobacter typing, food microbiology
Middlesbrough	+	+	+	
Newcastle, R	+	+	+	Syphilis serology, mycobacteria, staphylococcus phage typing, chlamydia
Norwich		+	+	
Nottingham	+	+	+	Legionella
Oxford, R	+	+	+	Group A streptococci, legionella
Peterborough		+	+	
Plymouth			+	
Poole		+	+	
Portsmouth	+	+	+	Brucella
Preston	+	+	+	Brucella, legionella
Reading	+	+	+	

Table 3 (*contd.*)

Laboratory	Diagnostic facilities for virology			Other reference services.
	EM	Culture	HBsAg	
Salisbury	+	+	+	
Sheffield, R	+	+	+	Haemophilus
Shrewsbury	+	+		
Southampton		+		
Stoke on Trent		+	+	
Taunton		+	+	Farmers' lung serology
Truro			+	
Watford			+	
Wolverhampton			+	
Cardiff, R	+	+	+	Group A streptococci
Carmarthen	+	+	+	
Conwy/Rhyl	+	+		
Swansea	+	+	+	Toxoplasma, diphtheria bacilli

R, regional laboratory.

space was such, however, that in 1976 it was decided to move the laboratory to the area PHLS laboratory at Norwich, at least until the new Colindale laboratories were ready. The laboratory was first set up at a time when it seemed that mycoplasmas might be concerned in a variety of disease in man; as it turned out few species other than *M. pneumoniae* have proved to be of great importance and the laboratory has done a fair amount of work on the taxonomy of strains from animals.

In 1972 the DHSS indicated that support could be made available for two additional reference laboratories, one for microbiology quality control, and one for work in support of chemotherapy: the intended functions of the latter were never very clear. A PHLS committee had been exploring methods for quality control for some time, and in 1974 a small laboratory was opened to take over the work of the committee (see p. 138). In 1979 the Microbiology Quality Control Laboratory was merged with the Standards Laboratory to form the Division of Microbiological Reagents and Quality Control.

The range of reagents produced by the Standards Laboratory for Serological Reagents increased dramatically as the range of diagnostic virology increased. Although the production of many bacterial reagents for use outside the PHLS had been transferred to the Wellcome Foundation in 1964, the laboratory continued to supply these reagents to PHLS laboratories. The laboratory was hard pressed during the mid-1970s to produce sufficient rubella antigen for the serotesting of women considered for vaccination; it also took responsibility for testing and distributing the commercial reagents used in tests for hepatitis B antigen and antibody. There were many discussions on the possibility of abandoning all production of reagents that were available in adequate quality from commercial sources; this would have released resources for the development of new or better reagents, and for the quality control of commercial reagents and media. The area laboratory directors, however, were always antagonistic to any suggestion that the Standards Laboratory should cease production of any reagent, holding that the quality and continuity of supply of commercial reagents could not be relied upon; possibly if regular quality control of such reagents could be established first there might be a change of heart, and one of the objectives of the newly constituted division was to increase the range of such work.

Two other laboratories were opened at Colindale during the decade. The Leptospirosis Reference Laboratory had been constituted in 1964 and had been housed at the London School of Hygiene and Tropical Medicine; in 1973 it was moved to a laboratory in the grounds of Colindale Hospital. In the same year the Bacterial Metabolism Research Laboratory was set up, also in the grounds of Colindale Hospital; it comprised a small research team who came with me from St Mary's Hospital Medical School to continue research that seemed to us of great public health importance, into the possible role of bacteria, in the gut or elsewhere, in the etiology of cancer.

Outside Colindale, the Tuberculosis Reference Laboratory at Cardiff was, after the retirement of Dr J. Marks in 1977, incorporated in the regional PHLS laboratory as the Mycobacterium Reference Unit. A great part of the work of the laboratory was first-line diagnostic work and the reference functions were more and more directed to mycobacteria other than *M. tuberculosis*. The laboratory continued to organize the quality control for drug susceptibility tests carried out by the regional laboratories for tuberculosis bacteriology, by now reduced to six in number.

Administrative developments at the Central Public Health Laboratory

It will be recalled that, from 1964, S.T. Cowan had combined the posts of Administrative Director at Colindale and Deputy Director of the Service. In 1967 he was succeeded in this combined post by J.C. Kelsey, who also continued to direct the small Disinfection Reference Laboratory. The combination of the two administrative posts, at Colindale and at the Park Crescent headquarters, was not very satisfactory and from 1971 the post of Administrative Director at Colindale was held in rotation by one of the reference laboratory directors. Many of the Colindale directors saw the individual reference laboratories as entirely independent units, and in no way part of an integrated central laboratory. They had indeed operated in this way for some years and there was no formal mechanism within the CPHL by which the work of the reference laboratories, or any deficiencies in the reference services, could be considered. Partly for this reason, but also because of the impending rebuilding of the central laboratory, the Board concluded, in 1974, that it would be desirable to re-establish the post of Director of the Central Public Health Laboratory. In the light of the Colindale directors' views, there was not surprisingly considerable debate on the terms of reference of the post, the Board wishing to see the Director of the CPHL in the role of leader and as manager of the CPHL budget, the directors mostly wishing to preserve nearly complete independence with direct and unfettered access to the Director of the Service. In the end a formula involving "co-ordinating and fostering maximum co-operation, but not directing the scientific work of the individual laboratories" was adopted.

After internal advertisement within the Service, Dr E.R. Mitchell, the director of the Nottingham PHLS laboratory, was appointed and took up the post in 1976; unfortunately illness meant that he had to give up the post in 1979. The Board reaffirmed its desire to appoint a director for CPHL, but not before Mr Sawyer – the Board Secretary – and I had conducted an exhaustive exercise in consultation with the staff of the laboratory. With the exception of the majority of the reference laboratory directors, staff of all other grades in the institution expressed a desire to see an overall director, although it has to be admitted that their reasons were various and in some cases unduly optimistic. At all events, the post was advertised and Professor A.A. Glynn, who held the chair of bacteriology at St Mary's Hospital Medical School, was appointed and took up his duties in the autumn of 1980.

The new Colindale

The DHSS had agreed in principle to the rebuilding of the CPHL on the adjacent Colindale Hospital site in 1969. Through 1970 and 1971 there were extensive consultations by the consultant architects, Robert Matthew, Johnson-Marshall and Partners, with the directors and staff of the reference laboratories to establish their current needs and future expectations. There then followed argument with the DHSS on the proposed area of the laboratories. The need to specify the use envisaged for individual areas at a very early stage in the Department's planning code inevitably led to the formulation of plans that were based on the expectations of the individual directors (none of whom was to be in post when building started) rather than to the design of non-specific multi-purpose laboratories. A restriction on the use of the 4 hectare site by the requirement of the Greater London Council that a substantial area should be left without building (to allow for the flooding predicted to occur once in 50 years) was an additional problem, and perhaps one that encouraged the architects initially to plan triangular laboratory blocks. Superimposed on the arguments concerning the detailed planning of the laboratories was an argument with the Department over the employment of management consultants; the Board rejected the idea, preferring to strengthen the Headquarters staff, despite a somewhat critical report on its management resources. In the light of all that followed this decision was almost certainly a mistake.

The "Stage A2" submission was sent to the Department in January 1974, but it was not until May 1975 that the Board heard that it could proceed to the next stage, subject to various discussions on large details, which in the event seem not to have been finally settled until 1978. It had been expected that a start could be made on site in the spring of 1977. However, the next stages of planning dragged on seemingly interminably. Although at the July 1977 meeting of the Board, Dr E.L. Harris, Deputy Chief Medical Officer at the Department of Health, was able to announce Ministerial approval, in principle, to the scheme going ahead, there was still much concern over the estimated cost, which had risen substantially. The Board itself was worried by the plans proposed for the ventilation of the laboratories, which had been developed with what seemed to be too slavish adherence to some features included in the brief as "desirable".

Negotiations, planning, replanning and cost-paring ground on, and although assisted by the appointment of a professional project manager (G.L. Rodham) in 1978, they were further slowed when the DHSS appointed a consultant engineer to make an independent appraisal of the structural engineers' plans. Despite initial claims that substantial savings would result from alternative plans, in the end these were shown to amount to no more than some £56,000. Eventually, after a discussion with the Secretary of State (Mr Patrick Jenkin) when he visited Porton in the autumn of 1979, the Board was given authority to proceed at a budget cost of £15 million (1979 prices).

However, problems were not yet over. The letter from the Department giving the authority was not clear that, despite some earlier indications to the contrary, the Board was expected to follow the capital developments code in full. Further there was some confusion over the pre-tender cost checks, and when the tenders were eventually

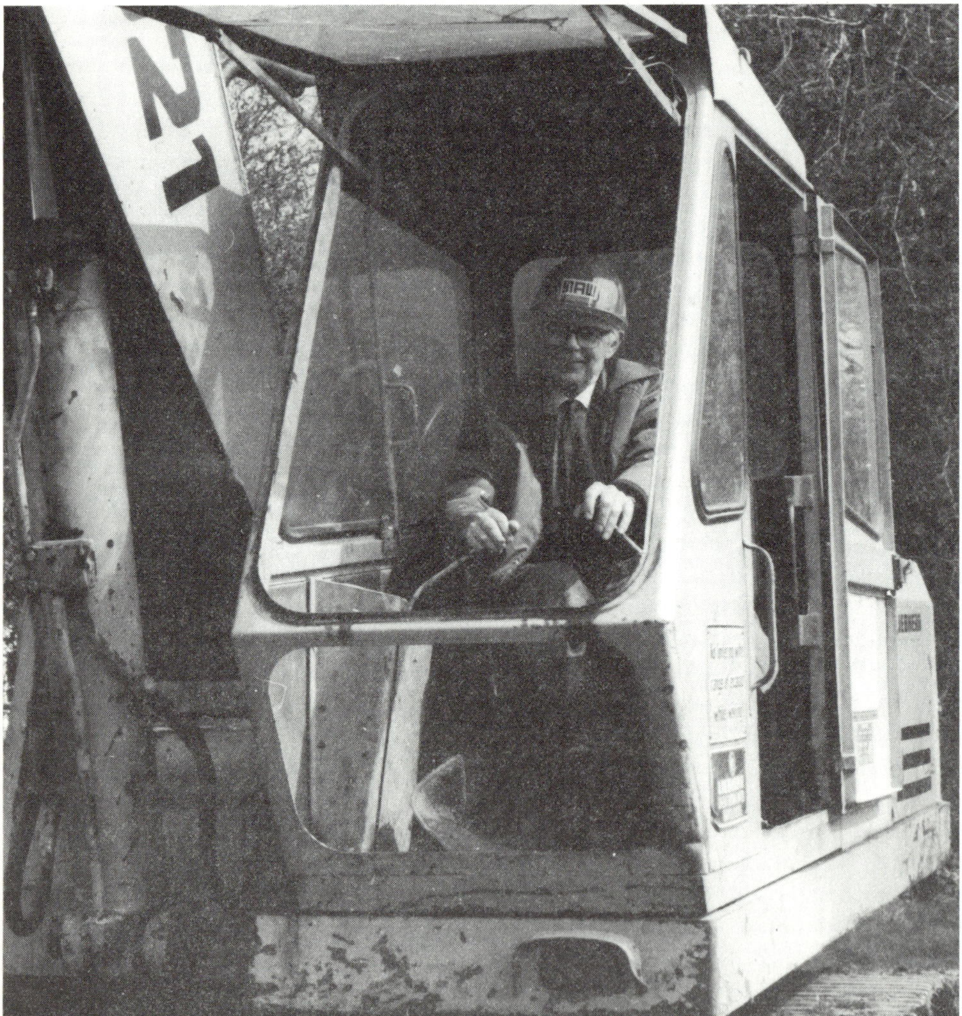

Figure 35 R.E.O.W. "digging the first sod" for the construction of the new Central Public Health Laboratory, April 1981.

received in June 1980, the lowest was £1.2 million over the budget cost. This led to great consternation at the "top of the office" in the DHSS, and in August a stop was put on all work on the project, fortunately soon modified to allow the continuation of the preliminary work on the ground that was already in progress. After the initial panic had subsided, a great effort was made by the design team, the headquarters office, DHSS officers and the contractors submitting the lowest tender (the Mowlem/Andrews-Weatherfoil joint venture) to achieve an acceptable reduction in the cost. This was eventually successful and the Board was able to accept the modified tender at the end of the extended time allowed by the contractors. I had the enjoyable task of digging a symbolic first sod with a JCB digger (Figure 35) in April 1981 (some few days after more professional diggers had moved in and cleared part of the site).

The Work of the Service, 1970–80

Epidemiology and information

From the beginning in the EPHLS the laboratory directors were encouraged to act also as field epidemiologists in support of the medical officers of health and it is probably fair to say that the epidemiological opportunities in the Service were among its particular attractions for recruits. At the same time Wilson (and indeed Scott too) had seen the need for including in the staff some who were primarily epidemiologists, and would almost certainly have appointed a number of "regional epidemiologists" had it not been for the opposition of the Society of Medical Officers of Health, and perhaps the Ministry. The Epidemiological Research Laboratory at Colindale was constituted in 1946 and rapidly became an important element in the Service, both in the support of routine and research activities in the field, and also in the organization of epidemiological information, particularly the Weekly Summary (from 1967 the *Communicable Disease Report*), and the annual reports on food poisoning.

In 1970 Howie published an important paper on the training of epidemiologists and the management of communicable diseases, and called for the establishment of a number of posts for regional epidemiologists within or closely associated with the PHLS. In the same year the Board agreed in principle to create a post for a trainee epidemiologist at Oxford. There was also a rather short-lived experiment in which an epidemiologist (D.L. Miller) was attached to the Exeter laboratory with, among other things, a remit to devise methods for the accurate measurement and assessment of the work of the laboratory. The experiment was short-lived because Miller was appointed Professor of Community Medicine at the Middlesex Hospital Medical School. Moore continued to attempt to assess the work of the laboratory (see Spencely *et al.*, 1979).

The outbreak of smallpox at the London School of Hygiene in 1973 (p. 161) was the subject of an Inquiry, chaired by Mr P.J. Cox, QC, and its report (Report, 1974), leaning heavily on evidence from Howie, recommended the setting up within the DHSS, and on the occurrence of smallpox, of a centre for the co-ordination of epidemiological inquiries and the control of the epidemic. It also recommended the establishment of a number of regional epidemiologist posts. When the DHSS eventually got round to considering the idea of a co-ordinating centre, it concluded that this should be on a permanent basis and not, as the report had suggested, a centre activated on the occurrence of an epidemic. At first it was proposed that it might be set up independently of the PHLS. This idea was fortunately soon abandoned and in 1976 the DHSS invited the PHLS Board to establish what became known as the Communicable Disease Surveillance Centre (CDSC); it was to be funded jointly by the DHSS and the

PHLS, and was to be separate from the Epidemiological Research Laboratory. The Board gladly accepted the invitation without, as it turned out, securing quite sufficient commitment from the DHSS to a joint funding that allowed for the rapid development of the Centre that ensued, following (and consequent on) the appointment of N.S. Galbraith as its director. CDSC took over the information services (the *Communicable Disease Report*) from February 1977, leaving the Epidemiological Research Laboratory to concentrate mainly on the surveillance of various immunization programmes and on hepatitis. Two regional epidemiologists were appointed, at Oxford in 1978 and at Manchester in 1979, and by 1980 the CDSC staff of epidemiologists had increased to four, with one in addition seconded from the DHSS, and two trainees in the senior registrar grade. The relationship between CDSC and the regional epidemiologists had not, by that time, been really satisfactorily worked out, but it seemed that such appointments would often be welcomed by medical officers for environmental health (whose predecessors had vetoed earlier proposals for such posts), while there was some suspicion on the part of laboratory directors who feared that they would be deprived of opportunities for field epidemiology. There was no doubt, however, that Galbraith had created an outstandingly successful unit in CDSC; some of its epidemiological investigations and analyses are mentioned later.

Medical officers of health, and their successors, had always been required to report serious outbreaks of infection directly to the DHSS (or Ministry), and in many cases medical officers from the Department had visited the area concerned, partly to assist the local medical officer of health and partly so that the Chief Medical Officer could be assured that proper methods for control were in hand. The medical officers from the Department were thus often investigating epidemics in which PHLS laboratories were also concerned, both in the laboratory and in the field. There were obvious opportunities for difficulties. It had always been the intention that CDSC should eventually take over this aspect of the Department's work, and after considerable delays the necessary Statutory Instrument was issued in February 1980. Thereafter it was to CDSC that the medical officers for environmental health had to report serious outbreaks, and it was CDSC's epidemiologists who were available to assist. The DHSS reserved to itself only epidemiological matters of international importance.

CDSC also initiated training schemes, both for individuals likely to become senior epidemiologists – Specialists in Community Medicine, Epidemiology, in the lingo of the discipline – and also for individuals aspiring to other posts in community medicine that might have responsibilities for communicable diseases.

In 1972 and 1973 the Staff Committee reviewed the scope and use of the *Communicable Disease Report* and considered (but rejected) the possibility of including information on tuberculosis and venereal diseases in it. The committee also returned to the vexed question of its confidentiality; the *Communicable Disease Report* had, at last in 1968, been made available to medical officers of health, but it was still considered inappropriate to make it an open publication, for fear of compromising some of the sources of information. A revised format for the *Communicable Disease Report* was introduced in 1974, and after CDSC took over the responsibility for it, the policy was to give it more of the character of a news-sheet and to reduce the extent to which "raw data" were included, in favour of more tabulations. The tradition of including accounts of epidemics was continued but there was a considerable increase in the number of analyses and short reviews of epidemiological situations, many of which were later published in the *British Medical Journal*. Another development was the production of joint reports on sexually transmitted diseases (with the academic department at the Middlesex Hospital Medical School) and on tuberculosis – two areas that had been long under-represented in the *Communicable Disease Report*.

CDSC also strengthened the PHLS's relations with the Animal Health Division of the Ministry of Agriculture, Fisheries and Food (MAFF), a veterinary epidemiologist from MAFF being attached part-time from April 1979. A nurse also worked part-time in the Centre for some time.

The question of the confidentiality of the *Communicable Disease Report* was raised once more, in 1980, this time after some protests from the medical correspondent of one of the daily papers. After discussion it was still felt that, despite a weekly circulation of 4000 copies, the *Communicable Disease Report* should not be issued as a public document, and should not be quoted publicly without permission from CDSC. The argument was, as previously, that much of the information included in the publication was gathered by laboratories operating under normal medical confidentiality rules, and that some information might be withheld if open publication were to be the rule. The worries of the press were accommodated by having one of the press officers of the DHSS attend the weekly meetings at which the content of the *Communicable Disease Report* is discussed, so that information could be made available to the press in appropriate circumstances.

The CDSC, after a temporary sojourn in a Portakabin on the CPHL site, was at first accommodated in an extension at the back of the headquarters office; a purpose-built unit on an adjacent site was finished in 1980 and formally opened by Sir Henry Yellowlees, the Chief Medical Officer, on 11 July 1980. After the ceremony he was presented with a miniature replica of the Broad Street pump, made famous by one of the first medical epidemiologists, John Snow.

From 1973 the Annual Reports of the PHLS included a chapter summarizing interesting features of the communicable diseases observed during the year; these were prepared by the Epidemiological Research Laboratory until 1976, and subsequently by CDSC. Quarterly contributions are published in *Community Medicine*, and from 1979 the annual report from the Office of Population, Censuses and Statistics on communicable diseases has been a joint publication with CDSC, which has contributed tabulations based on laboratory data.

Surveillance of immunization programmes

The Epidemiological Research Laboratory developed studies to monitor the effects of the national immunization programmes. The poliomyelitis survey has already been mentioned (p. 103); all reported cases are followed up to determine the vaccination history of the patient and contacts and the Virus Reference Laboratory tests any strains of poliovirus isolated from patient or contacts for marker characteristics that may indicate whether or not the strain is derived from the vaccine. For a long time reliance had to be placed on growth-temperature differences; the more satisfactory methods based on oligonucleotide mapping and specific antibody neutralization tests became available later.

The measles vaccine surveillance was based on the continued observation of some 20,000 children vaccinated in 1964–5; it was designed primarily to discover whether the immunity induced by the vaccine given in infancy was lasting, which it certainly seems to have been. Separate studies were made to measure reactions to the vaccine.

The national whooping cough vaccination programme was started after the PHLS/MRC studies had shown its potential benefit; the failure of some vaccines to generate adequate protection in the 1960s was revealed by PHLS studies (p. 114) and the doubts raised in the early 1970s on safety and efficacy called for renewed activity by the Epidemiological Research Laboratory. It was no longer possible to compare vaccinated children with randomly selected unvaccinated controls, but the less direct (and less convincing) methods used indicated that current vaccines were giving good protection. It was even more difficult to find thoroughly convincing methods of measuring the incidence of reactions to the vaccine, particularly the one type of reaction that is of real concern – the encephalopathy with severe neurological sequelae. Some studies made in the North-West Thames area contributed to the general conclusion that serious reactions are exceedingly rare.

The Epidemiological Research Laboratory has also had a long-term programme in which the tuberculin conversion rate induced by various batches of BCG is estimated each year.

The PHLS surveillance of influenza is described elsewhere (p. 156), and mention is also made elsewhere of observations on the prevalence of antibodies to rubella in women of child-bearing age (p. 159).

Monographs

In 1971 Howie proposed to the Staff Committee that members of the Service should be invited to write a series of short monographs which could summarize technical methods and other topics on which the PHLS had acquired special knowledge and expertise. Many members regretted the loss of the Monthly Bulletin of the PHLS and DHSS which had, during the 27 years of its publication, provided a useful vehicle for short technical accounts; it had ceased publication in 1967. Although the proposed scope of the monograph series was different, the idea was greeted with enthusiasm and the first three volumes were published in 1972. Others had a longer incubation period but by 1980 a total of 15 monographs had been issued (Table 4).

Quality control

Quality control, quality assessment, proficiency testing – various names have been applied to the activity involving the distribution of real or simulated specimens for laboratories to examine to test their skill in isolation or identification of microbes, or in estimation of antibody titre or antibiotic susceptibility. This was one of the growth industries of the 1970s. The PHLS Staff Committee set up a subcommittee in 1970, with R. Blowers as its chairman, which, in collaboration with Dr E. Joan Stokes and Dr

Table 4 PHLS monographs published, 1972–80

Monograph no.	Title
1	*Laboratory Diagnosis of Venereal Disease*
2	*The Use of Chemical Disinfectants in Hospitals*
3	*Anaerobic Bacteria*
4	*The Distribution and Identification of Non-fermenting Bacteria*
5	*Laboratory Methods 1* (incorporating articles on Elek's test of toxigenicity of corynebacteria; the isolation and identification of *Listeria monocytogenes*; the culture and identification of mycobacteria; infectious mononucleosis; isolation of lactobacilli from the genital tract)
6	*The Prevention of Laboratory Acquired Infection*
7	*Preservation of Bacteria, with Notes on Other Micro-organisms*
8	*Isolation of Salmonellas*
9	*The Trichomonads*
10	*The Bacteriological Examination of Urine: Report of a Workshop on Needs and Methods*
11	*The Vibrios*
12	*Basic Serodiagnostic Methods for Diseases Caused by Fungi and Actinomycetes*
13	*The Laboratory Diagnosis of Toxoplasmosis*
14	*Benchbook on Brucella*
15	*Isolation and Identification of Ringworm Fungi*

C.L. Greenbury, organized the distribution of some 86 test specimens to PHLS and to 26 hospital laboratories, to test their ability to isolate and recognize pathogenic bacteria and to do reliable antibiotic susceptibility tests. In 1974 the PHLS Microbiology Quality Control Laboratory was established in a small laboratory at Neasden Hospital, which had previously served as a sub-laboratory for the Colindale Diagnostic Reference Laboratory, and later for the PHLS laboratory at the Central Middlesex Hospital. Dr P.B. Crone was appointed director and with a very small staff he was able, in the first 16 months, to arrange the distribution of 50 specimens; by December 1975 a total of 287 laboratories in the British Isles (Scotland, Northern Ireland and Eire have participated in this exercise) were receiving specimens. In 1981, a total of 542 laboratories (415 in the UK) were taking part and 100 specimens were distributed. The PHLS Quality Control Laboratory was, from the start, recognized as an integral part of the National Quality Assessment Scheme, although funded by the PHLS rather than directly from the Department of Health. Like the schemes for other disciplines, there is a panel of professional advisers who are able to provide guidance and assistance to laboratories identified as persistently poor performers.

In 1979 the Quality Control Laboratory was merged with the Standards Laboratory to constitute a Division of Microbiological Reagents and Quality Control, with Dr P.S. Gardner as director. The Standards Laboratory had been conducting quality control tests on its own reagents, as well as on those made by the Wellcome Foundation, and the intention was to widen the scope of this testing to more reagents and to culture media, as well as to increase the scope of the specimens sent to the participating laboratories.

Other reference laboratories have had more informal arrangements for quality assessment: the Streptococcal Reference Laboratory organized an international comparison of serotyping in 1964–5; the Staphylococcal Reference Laboratory had also organized national and international comparisons of phage typing from 1957; the Tuberculosis Reference Laboratory made comparisons of the results of drug susceptibility tests carried out by the regional tuberculosis laboratories; and the Food Hygiene Laboratory participated in international trials of methods for the isolation of salmonellas from food.

Laboratory safety

The 1970s saw what amounted at times to an almost hysterical obsession with the problems of laboratory safety. There were good reasons for concern but not for hysteria. The 1973 outbreak of smallpox had originated in a laboratory infection; the Cox report on the outbreak recommended the establishment of a permanent committee to designate a list of hazardous pathogens, and to draw up regulations to govern laboratories handling them. The DHSS responded by setting up a working party, chaired by Sir George Godber, which soon discovered that a quite surprisingly large number and variety of institutions had stocks of dangerous pathogens. The committee's report (Report, 1975) offered a code of practice for the handling of the pathogens thought to be the most dangerous, based rather closely on the technique used at the Ministry of Defence's Microbiological Research Establishment at Porton Down. The Godber committee was followed by another DHSS working party, chaired by Howie, which was charged with constructing a code of practice for clinical laboratories.

In parallel with all this was the recognition of Lassa fever and the death of a number of hospital and laboratory workers in Africa and the USA from it; and simultaneously the molecular biologists' efforts to raise and later calm a hurricane of concern over the possible horrors of genetic engineering (see Williams, 1981).

The earlier PHLS interest in laboratory safety, particularly in relation to tuberculosis, has been mentioned above (p. 76) and in 1970–1 there were several discussions on improvements to the PHLS safety cabinet, including the introduction of an air-flow indicator utilizing a ping-pong ball. The realization that there were some potential hazards from the operation of centrifuges stimulated the setting up a subcommittee on their installation and operation. The need for laboratory clothing with greater protective capability than the conventional open-fronted coat led to the re-invention of a back-opening gown, originally used by Delépine in Manchester University. And there was the first indication of a need to appoint laboratory safety officers.

After the publication of the report of the Cox inquiry, a subcommittee was constituted to consider its implications for the PHLS laboratories offering diagnostic facilities for smallpox. When the Godber working party's report was published in 1975, it was clear that none of these laboratories could conform to the Porton-based recommendations for the handling of category A pathogens, but the Godber report had indicated that special attention needed to be given to diagnostic laboratories, and when the Chief Medical Officer's committee considered the laboratory requirements for handling material from patients in whom Lassa fever was one of the possible diagnoses, the smallpox laboratories were designated for the purpose.

In parallel with the deliberations of the Howie working party (which included in its membership J.E.M. Whitehead, then Deputy Director of the Service, and C.H. Collins, a senior technical officer in the Dulwich PHLS laboratory), the PHLS had its own safety committee which produced, in 1976, a general guide to laboratory safety. In addition, R.J. Henderson, the director the Worcester laboratory, was given the task of visiting all PHLS laboratories to advise on their structure, arrangements and safety precautions. These visits were undoubtedly of great value and were welcomed by the laboratories. But no sooner had Henderson reported on his surveys than the Howie code of practice was published (some many months after its contents had first been "leaked") and its requirements called for a further review of the laboratories' arrangements and equipment. It was estimated that to conform with all the code's requirements would have cost £570,000, though doubtless some "betterment factor" was included in the respective directors' estimates of their needs.

Meanwhile the Health and Safety Executive had started its programme of laboratory visits, initially adopting a policy seemingly calculated to antagonize laboratory directors by using the Howie code as the bible for the inspectors before it had been published. Their justification was that the inspectors had little or no experience of clinical laboratories, and what better guidance could there be than a code of practice produced by such a well qualified working party? The inspectors' zeal also led them to impose a formal veto on work with category A pathogens at Colindale, pending the completion of various structural alterations. Very fortunately for everyone – patients, clinicians, microbiologists and the inspectors – there were no suspect cases of smallpox, Lassa fever, or rabies while the veto was in operation.

The construction of a maximum security laboratory at Colindale was agreed in 1976; it was to be a totally separate building with its own air supply and filtered air effluent, as well as self-contained sterilizing plant for fluid effluent and a double-ended autoclave for getting material in and out. After inevitable difficulties with the ventilation system resulting from the need to have, within the room, extract-ventilated safety cabinets, the laboratory was finally commissioned in 1979. It was to be used for examining material from patients whose differential diagnosis included viral haemorrhagic fever, malaria, typhoid fever and so forth; the cultures for the haemorrhagic fever viruses were made at Porton. The Colindale laboratory also had a more regular use in the testing of rabies vaccine.

In the light of the possibility, as it seemed in 1976, of the closure of the diagnostic facilities at Porton, the PHLS Board agreed to construct special pathogen laboratories at Leeds, Liverpool, Birmingham and Cardiff. The first three were built and equipped with the totally enclosed train of safety cabinets similar to that developed at Porton. The complexity of the construction and various other factors resulted in astounding delays and by 1981 none of them was yet functional.

In the meanwhile the subcommittee on laboratory centrifuges designed and tested sealable buckets for the spinning of infectious material and the subcommittee on laboratory autoclaves had revealed the unsatisfactory operation of many autoclaves, as ordinarily used, and the unexpectedly long time that laboratory autoclaves ought to be allowed to cool before being opened. A system for direct air replacement by steam was devised by Mr Everall, in the Shrewsbury laboratory, and was incorporated in the specification for laboratory autoclaves drawn up by the subcommittee; prototypes were constructed for testing in 1980.

Computers and automation

The National Collection of Type Cultures (NCTC) had first become involved in the use of a computer to assist in the identification of bacteria around 1964, and from 1965 the Ministry had provided research funds to support a "Computer Trials Laboratory" under S.P. Lapage, who had succeeded Cowan as Curator of the NCTC in 1964. Computer matrices were constructed for the identification of Gram-negative bacilli and the laboratory offered a diagnostic service for bacteria of medical importance not identified by conventional methods. By 1974, 4027 strains had been received from 290 laboratories. The Computer Trials Laboratory was merged completely with the NCTC in 1978.

Lapage and his colleagues did a considerable amount of work on the theory and practice of numerical taxonomy (Lapage *et al.*, 1973; Hill, 1974) and diagnostic matrices have now been constructed to permit the computer-aided diagnosis of several different groups of bacteria, based on the strains deposited in the Collection or sent for identification – not always, of course, a random sample of the whole bacterial population. The use of a computer for generating reports and epidemiological information from routine diagnostic laboratory work was explored in the Norwich laboratory and elsewhere.

At the NCTC and elsewhere studies were made of mechanized or automated methods, and of other ways of improving or accelerating bacterial identification. Thus Taylor examined the possibilities of direct immunofluorescent staining methods, and various laboratories tested the application of enzyme-linked immunosorbent assay (ELISA). Ferguson and Tearle (1977) in the Luton laboratory used gas chromatography for the diagnosis of meningitis and of some anaerobic infections, while Johnston and others (1976) at Oxford looked at methods for mechanizing the counting of bacteria in urine and for antibiotic susceptibility testing, and Shipp and Rowe (1980), at Colindale, described one for salmonella typing.

The electron microscope became a very important part of the laboratories' diagnostic equipment. By 1976, 18 of the regional and area laboratories had their own microscopes and 13 others had ready access to instruments; their principal use was in diagnostic virology and in particular, during the late 1970s, in seeking virus particles in the faeces of patients with non-bacterial gastro-enteritis.

The PHLS played an important part in the organization of the 1976 International Symposium on Rapid Methods and Automation in Microbiology.

The National Collection of Type Cultures celebrated its 50th anniversary in 1971 with the publication of a history of its first 50 years, and a review of its current activities. Its main function is of course receiving, verifying and preserving strains of bacteria (and for a time bacteriophages), and the complementary function of issuing bacterial strains to research workers and others; in 1978, for example, the NCTC issued 7596 cultures, and freeze-dried a total of 107,622 ampoules. It had in addition a substantial research programme in bacterial taxonomy, apart from the computer work already mentioned. Much of this originated with groups of bacteria sent for identification and the recognition of clusters of taxonomically similar strains; in 1979 studies were made of various species of *Flavobacterium, Pseudomonas* and *Citrobacter*. Research has also been carried out on new methods for identifying bacteria, such as DNA analysis.

The Infections in the 1970s

Food poisoning

Whereas in the decade to 1969 we seemed to experience an almost steady state as far as developments in the field of food poisoning and other diarrhoeal diseases were concerned, with little overall increase in incidence until 1969 and the discovery and control of only a few new routes of salmonella infection, the 1970s were to see several important developments.

Around 1971 there were a number of outbreaks of acute gastro-intestinal illness characterized by violent vomiting attributable to the consumption of fried rice from Chinese take-away shops. The pathogen was shown to be *Bacillus cereus*. The Food Hygiene Laboratory collated these studies (Mortimer and MacCann, 1974; PHLS, 1976*a*) and worked on schemes for typing the bacilli (Gilbert and Parry, 1977) and on the toxic factors. It was evident that the fried-rice outbreaks had quite a different symptom pattern from the *B. cereus* diarrhoea previously recognized in Northern Europe. The bacilli were probably naturally present in the rice and their spores survived the cooking, to allow growth and toxin production during a period when the cooked rice was stored before frying.

Vibrio parahaemolyticus had been known for some time in Japan as a food-poisoning pathogen derived from seafood. Studies in the Truro laboratory showed that the vibrios were fairly common in seafood on sale in Britain (Barrow and Miller, 1972); the first food-poisoning incident recognized in Britain was recorded by the Poole laboratory in 1973 (Hooper *et al.*, 1974). Further outbreaks of illness have been very rare.

A third "new" bacterial cause of acute gastro-intestinal illness – *Campylobacter jejuni* – came sharply into the limelight after Skirrow's (1977) report in which he showed that, given appropriate technical methods, campylobacters could be isolated from the faeces of a substantial number of the patients suffering from acute diarrhoea who yielded no other pathogen. The appropriate techniques were rapidly adopted by the area laboratories and it was soon clear that an enormous number of cases of gastro-enteritis could now be given an etiological label; by 1981 the number of reports of campylobacter infections in the *Communicable Disease Report* exceeded that for salmonellas. Many laboratories set about investigating possible sources and modes of transmission; several dramatic incidents in which unpasteurized (either by intention or by mistake) milk was evidently the vehicle (Robinson *et al.*, 1979) demonstrated that campylobacters could be food-borne, but the nature of other pathways of spread had not yet been elucidated by 1980.

"Winter vomiting disease" is an ill-defined entity that has excited interest from time to time over the years and indeed the Reading laboratory carried out some studies around 1950 which suggested that even bread might sometimes be the vehicle of spread of some unknown agent. Later, American workers reported the transmissibility of a similar disease by means of faecal filtrates. The first good evidence for a viral origin for winter vomiting disease in Britain came from Dr Suzanne Clarke and colleagues who reported in 1972 on some volunteer tests carried out with extracts from faeces collected in 1963 and 1964 in a study by the PHLS Committee on Non-bacterial Gastro-enteritis. One extract produced symptoms in 21 of 26 volunteers, and faeces from one of these inoculated individuals was able to produce illness in another volunteer, thus demonstrating serial propagation, although at the time no direct evidence of a virus could be obtained. The disease produced was very similar to that due to the Norwalk agent studied in the USA. What may well have been the same agent was found in material from another school outbreak (Appleton *et al.*, 1977), revealed by immune electron-microscopy to have characteristics of a picornavirus, but to be antigenically different from the Norwalk agent. Caul and Clarke (1975) in the Bristol laboratory reported the electron microscopic detection of coronaviruses in material from three outbreaks of non-bacterial gastro-enteritis, with propagation of the virus in one case. Shortly after this Appleton and Pereira (1977), working in the Virus Reference Laboratory, demonstrated, also by electron microscopy, small round virus-like particles in the faeces of many of victims of a very large outbreak of gastro-enteritis that followed the consumption of cockles at a number of formal dinners in London at Christmas 1976.

In 1973 Flewett and his colleagues, working in the Birmingham Regional Virus Laboratory (not part of the PHLS but closely associated with the Birmingham PHLS laboratory), had described the rotavirus diarrhoea of infants. The infection had to be diagnosed by electron microscopy of faeces. By 1975 most PHLS laboratories had, or had access to, electron microscopes, and the evident importance of rotavirus infection in infants stimulated many to search faecal samples for different viruses, which were often found, and could sometimes be regarded as significant.

These new enteric pathogens were additions to the list of agents implicated in gastro-enteritis, not replacements. Salmonellas flourished. *S. typhimurium* maintained its place as the single most common serotype but the most dramatic feature of the salmonella scene was the rise to epidemic numbers of various other serotypes (Lee, 1974).

The increasing interest in salmonella contamination of animal feedstuffs has already been mentioned (p. 108) and several surveys were reported. For example, a collaborative study with Danish workers (PHLS *et al.*, 1972) revealed salmonella contamination of 23 per cent of samples of meat and bone-meal destined for animal feedstuffs. The widespread distribution of such feedstuffs resulted in the establishment of endemic infection in many of the herds and flocks of food animals and birds. A dramatic example of this mode of transmission was provided by the epidemic of *S. agona*, which was a very rare serotype in Britain until May 1970, when a few food-poisoning incidents attributable to poultry or pork were observed. Thereafter the number of *S. agona* incidents rose very fast: there were 232 incidents of human infection reported in 1971 and 620 in 1972, when it was the second commonest serotype. It was probably introduced in a consignment of fish-meal imported from Peru, and a similar pattern of spread was observed at much the same time in the USA and in several European countries. In subsequent years there were other, almost equally impressive, country-wide distributions of particular serotypes, such as that due to *S. senftenberg* in 1976, and the epidemic due to *S. hadar*, which increased the number of recorded isolates from 99 in 1974 to 2425 in 1978, the source of infection being nearly always turkeys or other poultry. A long-running although less extensive example was that reported by Payne and Scudamore (1977) of 185 cases of *S. enteritidis*, occurring over a period of eight years and all traceable to one turkey-breeding establishment.

Anderson had extended the research work of the Enteric Reference Laboratory into the genetics and molecular biology of the salmonellas, and the combination of classical serotyping with precise identification of the R-factors and transfer factors mediating antibiotic resistance provided superb tools for the characterization of strains and the tracing of their spread (Anderson *et al.*, 1978). McConnell and colleagues (1979) examined 89 strains of *S. wien* resistant to a range of antibacterial agents, and isolated in Britain and six other countries during 1970–7; they found that 85 per cent carried the same pair of plasmids, and they postulated that a clone had arisen in Algeria and subsequently spread across Europe. More recently Threlfall and others (1980) demonstrated the development of a whole series of drug-resistant strains among clones of salmonellas isolated from cattle.

The increase in poultry consumption that characterized the 1960s and 1970s was associated with a switch from other meats to poultry as the principal vehicle of salmonella food poisoning (McCoy, 1975) with, towards the end of the period, a considerable number of outbreaks due to turkeys – especially the large turkeys provided for weddings and large dinner parties. These and many other outbreaks were often traced to their source only by the concerted efforts of a number of laboratories working in collaboration with environmental health officers and sometimes the veterinary investigation laboratories.

A large outbreak of paratyphoid fever in Yorkshire, where the first isolation was from a cow, but where it was eventually shown that the cow probably became infected by drinking water polluted by a chronic human carrier, revealed some of the limitations of the powers of the veterinary authorities to investigate situations involving a risk to human health. The extent to which food-animals were being found as the source of salmonella infection in man was an important factor in leading the Ministry of Agriculture, Fisheries and Food to bring in the Zoonoses Order in 1977 and to establish local liaison committees which, it was hoped, would bring together the veterinary laboratories with environmental health officers, medical officers for environmental health and the public health laboratories. The joint PHLS/MAFF committee, originally constituted in 1962 (although a number of informal meetings had been held previously), was enlarged and renamed the Zoonoses Panel. It continued to provide a valuable forum for the exchange of information on the laboratory and field studies of the zoonoses, particularly salmonellosis; the provincial liaison committees varied greatly from one another in their achievements.

Two other general features of the salmonella scene deserve mention. There were a striking number of epidemics of salmonella infection in hospitals; for example, 53 were recorded in 1974. Although some were certainly examples of food poisoning, many were not, and case to case infection must have occurred, an interesting contrast to the food-poisoning outbreaks in which secondary cases are exceedingly rare. There were also several salmonella outbreaks due to the consumption of unpasteurized milk; in 1978 the Chief Medical Officer noted that some 3 per cent of the population were thought to consume unpasteurized milk, and that this vehicle appeared to be responsible for 7 per cent of all salmonella infections. Although it had been hoped, in 1975, that the sale of unpasteurized milk would be prohibited by 1980, objections from farmers and others led to postponement. A valuable survey of the hazards of unpasteurized milk was published by the Communicable Disease Surveillance Centre in 1982.

Food poisoning attributable to the enterotoxin of *Staphylococcus aureus* had declined steadily from about 1962, but investigation of such cases as occur was greatly helped by the development of methods for identifying the toxin production by staphylococci and for detecting its presence in food (Gilbert *et al.*, 1972).

Interest in *Escherichia coli* as an intestinal pathogen, quiescent since the epidemics of infantile diarrhoea in the 1940s and 1950s (p. 65), was reawakened by American workers' discovery of two enterotoxins produced by *E. coli* and presumptive evidence of the pathogenic activity of the toxins in travellers' diarrhoea. The techniques for detecting the toxins were established in the Salmonella and Shigella Reference Laboratory and in the Food Hygiene Laboratory, and were used to test strains from infantile diarrhoea; no strain was found that produced either toxin. Subsequent work showed that some cases of diarrhoea in children are, in fact, due to enterotoxigenic strains but it seemed that other mechanisms must also be involved.

The physiological behaviour of the infant gut was investigated in the Luton laboratory in an attempt to discover factors that might be concerned in the predisposition of bottle-fed infants to gastro-enteritis; it was proposed that the important factors were the low lactose, high protein content and the high buffering capacity of cows' milk, which favour the growth of *E. coli* in the gut rather than the lactobacilli (Bullen and Willis, 1971).

A small number of outbreaks of *E. coli* diarrhoea in adults were recorded, including three due to enterotoxigenic strains from Caribbean cruise ships studied by Hobbs and colleagues (1976). The interest aroused by the discovery of the two toxins – LT and ST – produced by *E. coli* and their putative relation to travellers' diarrhoea stimulated renewed interest in the pathogenesis of *E. coli* infections; the Division of Enteric Pathogens commenced a study of the factors that enable the bacteria to stick to the gut mucosa.

One startling but happily unique incident occurred in 1978 when four individuals who had shared a meal of canned salmon developed botulism; two died. The Birmingham laboratory and the Food Hygiene Laboratory collaborated in demonstrating the botulinum toxin in the serum of all four patients and in the remnants of the salmon in the suspect tin, from which *Clostridium botulinum*, type E, was also recovered.

The Food Hygiene Laboratory, in addition to its work on the enterotoxins of *Staphylococcus aureus* and *Bacillus cereus*, and on the serotyping of *Clostridium welchii* and *Bacillus cereus*, made studies of the hazards associated with various catering methods, such as the thawing of 30-pound frozen turkeys.

In the early 1970s it looked as though there would be a great increase in the demand for tests to determine the bacterial content of foods, generated by Britain's accession to the European Economic Community; many continental European countries had adopted microbiological standards to which it was thought that we should have to conform. Fortunately the combined strength of the PHLS and the DHSS representatives in the meetings at Brussels were effective in convincing the authorities that there was, in most cases, no good justification for quantitative microbiological standards for foods, or qualitative microbiological examination of food handlers. The discussions were, however, a stimulus to the setting up of strong "food and environmental bacteriology" sections within the regional PHLS laboratories at Leeds and Manchester, and to an increased emphasis on the methodology of food bacteriology in several laboratories, as well as in the Food Hygiene Laboratory.

Typhoid fever

The start of the 1970s saw the incidence of typhoid fever reach its nadir: 125 notifications in 1971, and even then the proportion of indigenous cases was low, for 90 of the 125 were thought to have been imported. During the ensuing decade the incidence rose gradually, to 241 notifications in 1978, but the rise was entirely due to importation, latterly mostly from the Indian subcontinent. The Enteric Reference Laboratory typed virtually all the strains of *Salmonella typhi* isolated in Britain and also received many strains for typing from other parts of the world. When the first substantial epidemic of typhoid fever due to chloramphenicol-resistant bacteria occurred, in Mexico in 1972, the laboratory was able to apply the various techniques of molecular biology that it had established to the elucidation of the origins of the new strain (Anderson, 1975). The Mexican epidemic was due to a clone of typhoid bacilli harbouring the H_1 R-factor coding for resistance to chloramphenicol, streptomycin, sulphanilamide and tetracycline. The same R-factor had been recognized in strains of different phage type in India, Vietnam and Thailand during 1972–4 and, significantly, drug-resistant strains of *S. typhimurium* from patients in South-East Asia were shown also to harbour H_1 R-factors. Anderson considered that various strains of typhoid bacilli had independently acquired the chloramphenicol-resistance plasmid from non-pathogenic intestinal organisms such as *Escherichia coli*, and had been selected by the widespread and indiscriminate use of the drug in the countries of South-East Asia and in Mexico.

The Croydon epidemic of typhoid fever, in 1937, was attributable to the contamination of the water supply to the town by an employee who was a carrier; after this it was the general policy among water authorities to require laboratory tests of potential employees, and this policy had continued despite the enormous decline in the prevalence of typhoid fever since 1937. The PHLS Committee on the Bacteriological Examination of Water Supplies pointed out, in 1978, that the Croydon outbreak was the last in which a major piped supply had been concerned, and advised, in the light of the decreased prevalence of infection, that the routine bacteriological and serological examination of employees was no longer sensible; it recommended restricting such examination to individuals for whom there were some definite indications.

Hospital-acquired infection

By 1970 two-thirds of the PHLS's laboratories were providing full bacteriological services for general hospitals and were inevitably involved in studies of hospital-acquired infection; and the reference services for typing staphylococci, streptococci and Gram-negative bacteria also played a vital part in the investigation of small outbreaks. Many of these were briefly reported in the *Communicable Disease Report*. The largest area of research was still in relation to the airborne spread of infection, particularly staphylococcal, based on the Cross-Infection Reference Laboratory (later the Division of Hospital Infection). Much of this work relied on the acquisition of nasal carriage of staphyloccocci as a marker. Two studies were carried out early in the decade to explore further methods that might be used for patient isolation within general wards. In a study at St Bartholomew's Hospital a ward was divided into two sections and mechanically ventilated to reduce aerial transfer of bacteria. In the second, at Queen Elizabeth II Hospital, Welwyn, the effect of isolation in conventionally ventilated side-wards was studied. In neither case was there any reduction in the rate at which patients became nasal carriers of *Staphylococcus aureus* (Lidwell *et al.*, 1970, 1971). In contrast Selkon and his colleagues (1980) were able to control the dispersal of a methicillin-resistant staphylococcus by isolation of all patients infected with, or carrying, the strain in a mechanically ventilated isolation unit separate from the main ward area.

Laminar flow or, as it is better termed, unidirectional ventilation seemed to offer an alternative to solid walls for isolation, and might have great advantages in some areas such as an intensive therapy units. Lidwell and Towers (1972) explored this use and found that, although mechanically efficient, the patients nursed in the ventilated areas still acquired staphylococci at a rate similar to those nursed in the conventionally ventilated area. But the biggest study of the 1970s was that led by Lidwell in the new Greenwich District Hospital, which was totally air-conditioned. Sophisticated methods were devised to monitor not only the air-change rates but also the extent to which air and airborne particles, including bacteria, were exchanged between the different rooms and other areas of the ward. The monitoring system worked, at first, rather better than the ventilation and demonstrated the need for major adjustments. The work revealed that the spread of staphylococci from patients in one room to the air of another occurred to a greater extent than could be accounted for by air movement (Lidwell *et al.*, 1975). Taking all these studies together it seemed likely that the staphylococci were being conveyed from one patient area to another on nurses' clothing. This led to a further interest in the bacterial permeability of various fabrics used, or usable, for surgeons' and nurses' uniforms – a topic on which various PHLS laboratories had worked for some 20 years.

At the end of the decade Lidwell was to become a leading investigator in a very large multi-centre study of "ultra-clean air" in operating rooms used for hip-replacement surgery, with, for a change, a good indication that substantial protection was afforded.

The Staphylococcus Reference Laboratory conducted an 11-year survey of the strains of *Staphylococcus aureus* isolated from infected patients in a series of London hospitals, which was reviewed, under the title "Endemic staphylococcal infections in hospitals" (Parker *et al.*, 1974) in the context of earlier studies, including my own paper entitled "Epidemic staphylococci" (Williams, 1959). The change in adjective reflected not only a greater understanding of the pattern of staphylococcal behaviour in hospitals, but also the virtual disappearance of the phenomenon, seen in the 1950s, of the dramatic spread of particular, apparently unusually virulent, phage types.

Various developments in surgical practice have given opportunities for what used to be considered non-pathogenic bacteria to invade and cause disease: cardiac surgery has been particularly helpful to the coagulase-negative staphylococci. Phage typing schemes were developed for these bacteria in several places, and though technically much less satisfactory than the *S. aureus* scheme, have been of some epidemiological use, as for example in a long-running outbreak of infection in a cardiac surgery unit (Marples *et al.*, 1978).

The conventional wisdom of the past 15 or so years has been that, in the field of hospital-acquired infection, the staphylococcal menace has been replaced by a "Gram-negative" menace, even though a large PHLS study, published after the end of this survey, still revealed staphylococci as the single most common pathogen in surgical wound sepsis. But, certainly, an increasing variety of Gram-negative bacilli have been incriminated in outbreaks and sporadic cases of hospital infection. The Cross-Infection Reference Laboratory extended its terms of reference to pyogenic and septicaemic infections due to Gram-negative bacilli, other than those affecting the gut, and developed typing schemes to assist epidemiological study of several different species: first *Pseudomonas aeruginosa* (Wahba, 1965; Pitt and Bradley, 1975) and later *Serratia marcescens* (Pitt *et al.*, 1980) and *Enterobacter*. A *Klebsiella* typing service was developed in the Coventry PHLS laboratory.

Bassett (1971) analysed several common-source outbreaks due to Gram-negative bacilli, while outbreaks of bacteraemia due to contaminated transfusion fluids were studied at Plymouth and, by the Oxford laboratory, at Kettering. The possibility that pharmacy practices might be responsible for contamination of medicaments was investigated by a PHLS subcommittee set up in 1966 and by Joynson and colleagues (1975). Right at the end of the period covered by this review, the Oxford laboratory uncovered an important reservoir for *Legionella pneumophila* in hospital shower mixers, and also in hospital and hotel water supply systems and air-conditioning cooling units (Tobin *et al.*, 1981).

The serotyping of *Escherichia coli* was developed in the Salmonella Reference Laboratory primarily for the study of strains isolated from faeces of infants with diarrhoea. The typing service was never generally available for the examination of *E. coli* from other sources, although a few small investigations were reported (e.g. Bettelheim *et al.*, 1971).

Reference has been made elsewhere to studies of salmonella infections in hospitals; in the present context it is of interest to note that in 52 of 76 salmonella outbreaks in hospitals for which a "source" was recorded (in PHLS, 1980*a*) transmission was thought to be by some route other than food, but the alternative modes of spread of salmonellas have not been examined in the sort of detail used for staphylococci or the Gram-negative pyogenic organisms.

In the field of viral infections only hepatitis (p. 159) has been studied in any detail as a hospital-acquired infection, although there can be no doubt that respiratory virus infections are transmitted in hospital (see Sims *et al.*, 1981).

The lead given by Moore in introducing a plan for appointing a member of the nursing staff to monitor infections in hospitals was noted earlier (p. 112); by the 1970s very many hospitals had made such appointments, and in many cases these infection control nurses were actually based in the laboratory. A Staff Committee discussion in 1977 considered the ways in which laboratory workers could assist the nurses, who were, according to one speaker, dear to the heart of many directors. Both Moore and Galbraith served as President of the Infection Control Nurses' Association.

Legionnaires' disease

The first case of Legionnaires' disease recognized in England was identified by the Nottingham laboratory in 1977 (Macrae and Lewis, 1977), and in the following year the first isolation of *Legionella pneumophila* in the United Kingdom was reported by the Cambridge laboratory. The Standards Laboratory received type strains of the organism from the United States and prepared a formalized yolk-sac antigen for use in diagnostic serology; there was some evidence that this was less liable to give non-specific cross-reactions than the ether-killed antigen originally supplied by the US Centers for Disease Control, Atlanta (Taylor *et al.*, 1979). The diagnostic value of gas–liquid chromatography and mass spectroscopy in the identification of the bacterium was demonstrated in the Bacterial Metabolism Research Laboratory (Fisher-Hoch *et al.*, 1979). In a very short time, a survey by questionnaire assembled epidemiological data on 84 sporadic cases with onsets during January 1976–September 1978 (Bartlett, 1979). The importance of domestic water supplies as well as air-conditioning systems as reservoirs of legionellas soon became evident, though most of this work was reported after 1980.

Yersinia *infections*

Mair's studies of *Yersinia* infections continued to reveal the occurrence of mesenteric adenitis due to *Y. pseudotuberculosis* (260 cases between 1961 and 1978) and also showed what appeared to be a real rise in the frequency of *Y. enterocolitica* infections.

Urinary tract infections

Despite the very large number of specimens of urine examined in PHLS laboratories (1.6 million in 1979), relatively little research or development has been carried out on urinary tract infections. However, both at Plymouth and Portsmouth, the importance of coagulase-negative staphylococci and micrococci as urinary tract pathogens in young adult women was demonstrated, and at Portsmouth Maskell made a long series of studies in the less fashionable reaches of urinary tract infections, such as children, males and the urethral syndrome. The number of urines coming to the laboratory each day seem to make urinalysis an ideal subject for automation and Johnston, at Oxford, worked for many years to achieve a usable system, as did Human in Plymouth. The difficulty is that the standard screening methods for urine are now very rapid and simple, and until some technique to give a more or less instant answer can be devised, they are unlikely to be superseded.

Streptococcal infections

Infections with Group A haemolytic streptococci (*Streptococcus pyogenes*) have not generated much interest in Britain during the last 20 years, although there were still around 13,000 notifications of "scarlet fever" in 1970 (many of these were probably not streptococcal infections; Perks and Mayon-White, 1983), and isolated incidents of severe streptococcal infection are not infrequently reported. There was, however, a continuing research interest in *S. pyogenes* in the United States and the streptococcus reference section of the Cross-Infection Reference Laboratory continued its collaboration with American workers, directed particularly to the skin infections that are common in the tropics and which, in Trinidad, had been shown to cause a high incidence of acute glomerulonephritis. The "skin streptococci" usually belonged to serotypes different from "throat streptococci", and were initially often difficult to type. The epidemiological differences between skin and throat strains of streptococci stimulated a considerable amount of work on the various antigens and on the antibody response to infection. The "opacity factor" originally described in the Streptococcus Reference Laboratory in 1961 proved to offer a useful complementary method for type identification (Maxted *et al.*, 1972). It also became clear that there were differences in the antibody response in acute rheumatic fever and in glomerulonephritis; furthermore, after skin infections very little antistreptolysin-O is formed, though the antibody response to other extracellular antigen may be considerable; the significance of this difference is not yet apparent.

Around 1974 some laboratories noted an undue prevalence of *Streptococcus pyogenes* skin infections in workers in abattoirs; one particular type of streptococcus was found in a number of outbreaks, while being rarely isolated elsewhere. There was some indication that it might survive especially well on raw meat (Fraser *et al.*, 1977). The investigation also highlighted hygienic deficiencies that clearly offered the streptococci additional facilities for spread.

The Streptococcus Reference Laboratory continued to act as one of the three laboratories recognized internationally for the identification of new serotypes of *Streptococcus pyogenes*.

In the late 1960s there was a considerable increase in interest in human infections with Group B streptococci, particularly as a cause of septicaemia and meningitis in the newborn; some American work indicated an incidence approaching 3 per cent of live births. From anecdotal reports it seemed unlikely that the incidence was as high in Britain, but in 1976 a subcommittee was constituted to carry out a survey, in which 10 laboratories participated; this revealed an attack rate well below one per 1000 (Parker, 1979). In the meanwhile, Stringer and Maxted (1979), in the Streptococcus Reference Laboratory, had devised a phage typing method that proved of considerable use in studies to determine the origin of the infections in babies, and in particular the extent to which the infants' infections could be attributed to infection from the mother's vagina.

Our ability to classify the non-haemolytic streptococci was given a considerable impetus by an extensive taxonomic study carried out at St Mary's Hospital Medical School by G. Colman, who later joined the Division of Hospital Infection at Colindale. Parker and Ball (1976) developed Colman's methods and set out to classify a collection of 820 streptococci isolated from patients with endocarditis and other systemic infections; the 317 strains from endocarditis could all be allocated to recognized taxa. It was notable that dextran-forming species – *Streptococcus mutans, S. bovis* I, *S. sanguis* and some *S. mitior* – were particularly common in endocarditis, while *S. milleri* was prominent among strains from septic lesions in internal organs. The studies of *S. milleri* in particular emphasized the need to use several criteria for identification: 28 per cent of *S. milleri* strains have one or other of four Lancefield "group" antigens, while 25 per cent are β-haemolytic.

Gonorrhoea

The Chief Medical Officer's comments on gonorrhoea during the 1970s ranged from regret that we do not live in a "monogamous and sexually continent society" (in 1970, when there were 53,525 reported cases) to the assertion that the disease "continues to be controlled by the efficiency and co-ordination of all grades of staff in the clinics" (in 1976, when the number of cases was 58,444). In the middle of the decade the long-feared penicillinase-producing gonococci turned up, more or less simultaneously in Liverpool (Turner *et al.*, 1976) and London (Phillips, 1976; Wilkinson *et al.*, 1976); the Venereal Disease Reference Laboratory had been monitoring the resistance of gonococci for some years and continued this study after the penicillinase-producing strains appeared. For a few years very few more strains were seen, but in 1979 they reappeared, and the laboratory identified 61 penicillinase-producing strains among 355 sent for investigation.

Syphilis

Serological tests for syphilis continued to provide a good deal of work for the area laboratories (nearly 400,000 sera for diagnosis of "VD" were received in 1979) and the Venereal Diseases Reference Laboratory carried out confirmatory tests on some 21,000 sera from other centres. It and the Newcastle PHLS laboratory, together with the Regional Serology Laboratory at Manchester, provided the national service for the TPI (treponemal immobilization) tests.

Non-gonococcal urethritis

There was in this period a great increase in the number of cases of non-gonococcal urethritis and a considerable amount of research in various centres into its etiology. The principal contribution from the PHLS was Shirley Richmond's study, in the Bristol laboratory, of methods for isolating strains of chlamydia A, including the use of cytochalasin-treated McCoy cells (Sompolinsky and Richmond, 1974). She and some other PHLS laboratories investigated the possible role of chlamydias in urethritis. While at first there seemed to be some doubt as to their role as primary pathogens, in view of the frequency with which chlamydias are found in gonococcal as well as non-gonococcal urethritis (Richmond *et al.*, 1972), by 1978 it had become generally accepted that chlamydias are responsible for a substantial proportion of the cases of non-gonococcal urethritis and efforts were concentrated on developing routines that would make best use of laboratory facilities for detecting infection in women (Richmond *et al.*, 1980).

Tuberculosis

In relation to tuberculosis, the contribution to laboratory safety was mentioned earlier. The main thrust of the Tuberculosis Reference Laboratory was in the continued investigation of mycobacteria other than *M. tuberculosis*, culminating in a valuable scheme for their classification using methods available in clinical laboratories (Marks, 1972), supplemented by a scheme for the examination of *M. tuberculosis* and other mycobacteria by methods available in laboratories with restricted facilities, prepared at the request of the World Health Organization (Marks, 1976). More refined methods, such as lipid analysis, for reference laboratory work were also studied (e.g. Jenkins, 1981*a*). Jenkins (1981*b*) estimated that the annual number of infections in England and Wales, due to opportunist mycobacteria, might be around 200. The laboratory continued to co-ordinate the work of the six regional laboratories providing drug susceptibility testing services.

Tuberculosis steadily declined in incidence during the decade, from 11,280 notifications in 1970 to 8752 in 1980, and there was widespread speculation on the continued usefulness of BCG vaccination. Sharp reminders that the disease can still strike were offered by two outbreaks, in the investigation of which CDSC participated, that occurred in 1979 and 1980; in the former 108 children became infected, five having clinically evident tuberculosis, by what seemed surprisingly distant contact with a swimming-bath attendant. In the second, the source was a dentist.

Meningococcal meningitis

The early 1970s saw a sharp increase in the incidence of meningococcal meningitis which, in the light of substantial outbreaks in Brazil and in Finland, looked somewhat menacing; after rising to 1105 notifications in 1974 (from 494 in 1970 and 406 in 1965) the number of cases declined. The Manchester laboratory and the Standards Laboratory at Colindale provided a service for determining the serogroup (the majority being B with many fewer A and C) and the Manchester laboratory carried out surveys of sulphonamide susceptibility (only 6 per cent were resistant). The laboratory also studied the use of counter-current electrophoresis of cerebrospinal fluid for diagnosis (Abbott and Graves, 1972). Later, studies were also made of the protein antigens of the meningococci, which could be used to supplement the polysaccharide antigen typing, and might perhaps be useful as protective antigens (Jones and Eldridge, 1981).

Aseptic meningitis

"Aseptic" or non-bacterial meningitis has long been recognized as a clinical entity; the use of the now abundant facilities for the diagnosis of virus infections was by the 1970s able to provide a precise diagnosis in many cases. It also revealed how different viruses had periods of prevalence, and could thus virtually disappear from the scene for several years. In 1978 echovirus 11 was reported from 530 cases of meningitis and encephalitis; in 1974 echovirus 19 had been reported from 566 patients, about 60 per cent of those with symptoms recorded having had meningitis. The overall picture of viral meningitis and encephalitis for one year – 1979 – was reviewed by Noah and Urquhart (1980*a*), summarizing the reports to the Communicable Disease Surveillance Centre and the Communicable Diseases (Scotland) Unit; no fewer than 18,407 reports were received.

Influenza

The PHLS contribution to the study and control of influenza during the 1970s was concentrated largely on developing methods for surveillance and prediction of epidemics. After the substantial epidemic due to the Hong Kong virus in 1969–70, the Staff Committee discussed the methods available for case-finding, and in 1972 a joint subcommittee was set up with the Royal College of General Practitioners. A PHLS report (PHLS, 1975) summarized the schemes that had been devised and the results have been reported in a number of papers in later years. For a number of years from 1972 several laboratories collaborated, each recruiting a local general practitioner and medical officer of health to collect specimens and information, from a surveillance population in the region of 150,000. The practitioners agreed to collect nose and throat swabs from a sample of their patients with acute respiratory disease, thus enabling the calculation of a "virologically estimated influenza rate". In addition, statistics from a wider general practice population were available from the Royal College of General Practitioners, numbers of new sickness-benefit claims were available from the DHSS and numbers of deaths were available from the weekly returns to the Office of Population, Censuses and Statistics; and the number of virus isolations reported from PHLS and other laboratories were recorded in the *Communicable Disease Report*, and their antigenic make-up was examined in the Virus Reference Laboratory. The results of the first three years (PHLS, 1977) (Figure 36) covered a period of relatively low activity, the virologically estimated influenza rate exceeding 200 per 100,000 in only one week. The availability of laboratory results meant that good data were also available for infections due to the influenza B virus which, because it commonly affects children and causes very little serious illness, is unnoticed in the morbidity statistics for the adult population. The laboratory results for some 8800 isolates of influenza virus for 1968–76 were summarized by Pereira and Chakraverty (1977), and documented the change from the original Hong Kong virus, through some five H3N2 variants, and also changes in the prevalent B viruses.

Influenza is one of the infections that attracts interest in the press and speculation of the possibility of an epidemic during the next winter, or on the likely course of an epidemic already in progress, and some reliable supplement to the crystal ball as an

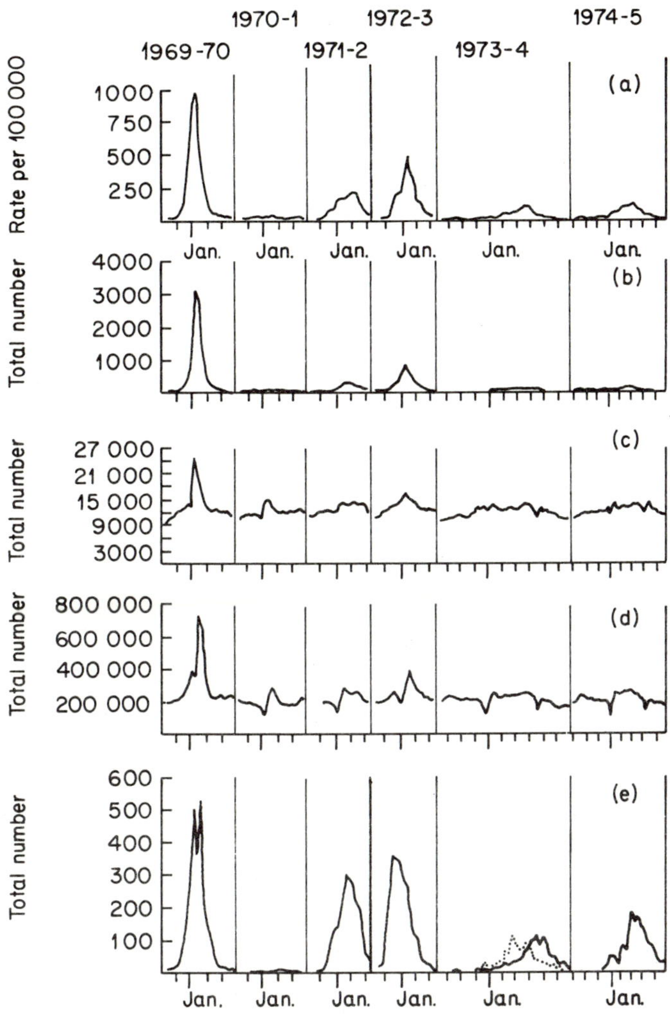

Figure 36 National influenza statistics, 1969–75. (a) Incidence of influenza in England and Wales, compiled from returns to the Royal College of General Practitioners; (b) deaths from influenza and influenzal pneumonia in England and Wales; (c) deaths from all causes in England and Wales; (d) new sickness-benefit claims (England, Wales and Scotland); (e) influenza virus isolations in England, Wales and Scotland, as reported in the *Communicable Disease Report* (———, influenza A; ······, influenza B). (Redrawn with modifications from PHLS, 1977.)

aid to prediction would be very valuable. Over the years during which detailed surveillance has been carried out, however, there have been a good many surprises and it cannot be said that confident prediction is yet possible. A very detailed analysis (Clifford *et al.*, 1977), applying regression techniques to the data available from morbidity and mortality statistics, laboratory findings and air temperature did appear to offer a reasonable estimate of the excess mortality attributable to influenza in any particular year. In years with substantial epidemics there appeared to be up to 27,570 excess deaths; in no year between 1967 and 1975 were they fewer than 1570.

Apart from the work on case-finding there were more general studies on the epidemiology of influenza: Pereira and colleagues (1972) studied the prevalence rates for antibodies to the current strains of virus and the use of these rates in the prediction of the value of vaccines.

From 1974 the DHSS medical officers had analysed the available surveillance data weekly during the winter seasons, and compared reported incidence with calculated "non-epidemic means" and "threshold levels" as a measure of epidemic prevalence. From the autumn of 1977 this influenza watch was taken over by the PHLS Communicable Disease Surveillance Centre and further refined. Weekly reports have been issued in the *Communicable Disease Report*, with more detailed summaries at appropriate intervals.

From 1948 the World Health Organization had recognized what had originally been Sir Christopher Andrewes' laboratory at the National Institute for Medical Research as the World Influenza Centre. In 1976 it was agreed that its successor, the WHO Collaborating Centre for Reference and Research on Influenza, should be run jointly by the PHLS Virus Reference Laboratory and the Virology Division of the National Institute for Medical Research. The Virus Reference Laboratory had responsibility for identifying the influenza viruses isolated in Britain and in some countries overseas.

The MRC Influenza Vaccine Trials Committee continued to study vaccination and the PHLS laboratories provided support. In addition the Epidemiological Research Laboratory carried out a trial among workers in the Post Office, and found some evidence of benefit (Smith and Pollard, 1979); on the other hand a long series of studies, by the Guildford laboratory, among the boys in Christ's Hospital School indicated that, overall, annual revaccination had no long-term advantage; revaccination with one strain did not increase protection, and vaccination with a later strain did not protect against subsequent challenge (Hoskins *et al.*, 1979).

Respiratory virus infections

Other respiratory virus infections were reported in increasing numbers as facilities for their diagnosis became available; the Annual Reports of the PHLS for 1973 onwards note some of the interesting findings each year. Unlike the enteric viruses there was no research group with a particular interest in respiratory tract viruses after the large collaborative study of the 1960s (Miller, 1973) had been completed and after the small Epidemiological Research Unit under Dr R.E. Hope Simpson at Cirencester had closed. Higgins, working in Cirencester, summarized the experience of that unit, and also produced evidence for the pathogenicity of the coronaviruses (Higgins, 1974). The pattern of rhinovirus infection in Britain was reviewed by Roebuck in 1976.

A collaborative study with university health physicians demonstrated the relevance of Epstein–Barr virus infection to infectious mononucleosis (PHLS, 1971) and there was a small continuing programme of laboratory research into the behaviour of Epstein–Barr virus and the antibody response to it, particularly the IgA response (Edwards and Woodruff, 1979).

From about 1967 many laboratories were able to seek respiratory syncytial virus, using direct immunofluorescent techniques that could give a very rapid answer.

Mycoplasma infections

Mycoplasma infections of the respiratory tract seem to occur every four years in country-wide epidemics, each lasting about two years: outbreaks were recorded in 1967–8, 1971–2, 1974–5, 1977–9, and again in 1981–2. At the peak of the 1977–9 outbreak over 450 cases were recorded in one four-week period from the laboratories contributing to the *Communicable Disease Report* and the Communicable Disease (Scotland) Unit (Noah and Urquhart, 1980*b*). The great majority of these infections were manifested in the lower respiratory tract – "atypical pneumonia".

Rubella

The DHSS rubella vaccination campaign was started in September 1970, initially confined to schoolgirls between their 11th and 14th birthdays. At that time there were not sufficient laboratory facilities for the antibody determinations that were considered essential before vaccine could be given to women of childbearing age. Several PHLS laboratories were investigating methods for serotesting, and by 1976 it was felt that there should be no serious difficulties in offering to test all women presenting for vaccination; the DHSS initiated a campaign to attract adult women. In 1977 the laboratories received more than 505,000 sera for rubella antibody tests, a figure that had risen to about 783,000 by 1980. Initially the tests were carried out by the haemagglutinin-inhibition method, using (in rather large quantity) antigen prepared in the Standards Laboratory. By 1978 it had become clear that the single radial haemolysis method would offer many advantages; a subcommittee was set up to conduct comparative tests and define a standard procedure (Russell *et al.*, 1978) and before long single radial haemolysis was being widely used, with great economy of material and time. Throughout this period, too, studies were being carried out on various methods for distinguishing IgG and IgM antibodies and their application in cases of the congenital rubella syndrome, and in women exposed to rubella during pregnancy. Cradock-Watson and colleagues (1976) demonstrated the advantage of the indirect immunofluorescent technique applied to sucrose-density fractions of sera.

Hambling (1980) reported the Leeds experience with some 150,000 antibody tests on women of childbearing age between 1971 and 1978 and found evidence that the childhood vaccination programme was having some effect in that the proportion of women who were seronegative declined from 11.3 to 7.7 per cent. As is known there are, however, still a large number of seronegative women becoming pregnant each year and at risk from infection; the DHSS has again launched an active campaign.

Hepatitis

A leading article in *The Lancet* in 1969 considered that outbreaks of hepatitis seemed to be inevitable in renal dialysis units; the work of the PHLS Virus and Epidemiological

Research Laboratories over the next 10 years was happily to show that this was not true. At the time when the association of Blumberg's Australia antigen (HBsAg) was demonstrated in 1968, renal units in Britain had suffered serious outbreaks of hepatitis in patients and staff, so there was strong pressure to provide a diagnostic service. In 1971 a total of 13 PHLS laboratories were designated hepatitis reference laboratories, available to assist hospital laboratories in their areas (although curiously they were never listed as such in the PHLS Directory); by 1973, PHLS laboratories were examining over 120,000 specimens a year for HBsAg. At the same time the Blood Transfusion Service was instituting tests for HBsAg on all donations and in some areas the PHLS was involved in this work, either in the first-line screening or in confirmation of presumptive carriers.

The subcommittee on the infection risks of haemodialysis, set up in 1967 and comprising individuals with experience in hospital-acquired infection, was particularly concerned with improvements in the hygienic precautions of dialysis unit practice. A prospective study of hepatitis in dialysis units, in which Sheila Polakoff in the Epidemiological Research Laboratory and Yvonne Cossart in the Virus Reference Laboratory played a leading part, was commenced in 1970. Previous pilot studies had shown a rising incidence of infections, and the association of the infections with HBsAg (Polakoff *et al.*, 1972). The study soon showed that the introduction of a patient who was already an antigen carrier was the most important source of infection for a unit, so that intensive screening for antigen in patients and staff constituted the first line of defence; it had to be supplemented by the treatment in isolation of known carriers and by the strengthening of measures against cross-infection. By 1972 (Polakoff, 1974) the incidence of hepatitis in patients had declined from 4.9 to 1.4 per cent, and in staff from 1.3 to 0.4 per cent. By 1973 these figures were further reduced to 0.3 and 0.1 per cent (PHLS, 1976*b*); in contrast some figures for renal dialysis units in the United States in 1972–4 indicated attack rates on patients of some 24 per cent and on staff of 11 per cent. Although screening of blood used for transfusion and of patients and staff was essential, a major contribution to control was seen as prevention of cross-infection within the unit by hygienic methods.

The issue of immunoglobulin for the prophylaxis of various infections has always been administered by the Epidemiological Research Laboratory at Colindale and from about 1973 studies were made of the use of hepatitis immunoglobulin (HBIG) in the prevention of hepatitis after accidental inoculation. This study was carried out in collaboration with an MRC committee and although no untreated control group was available, the conclusion finally reported in 1980 was that the prophylaxis was effective (MRC and PHLS, 1980).

The problems in dialysis units highlighted the risks for staff and an outbreak in Edinburgh had demonstrated that the risk extended to the laboratory, a fact confirmed by Grist's early report (Grist, 1975). This problem has been extensively debated, but largely outside the PHLS. The converse risk, that hospital staff may infect their patients, is one that clearly demanded the sort of nation-wide exploration for which the PHLS is well fitted, but because of the threat that might be posed by the discovery of symptomless carriage in a member of the hospital staff, early attempts to set up a study were foiled. It was not until after the recognition of eight cases of hepatitis among the patients operated on by one gynaecologist (PHLS, 1980*b*), that it was possible to get agreement to a surveillance scheme, still at the time of writing in progress.

The general increase in the application of tests for HBsAg during the 1970s led to much better understanding of the epidemiology of hepatitis B virus infections, in particular in relation to sexual, and especially homosexual, transmission, and to the excess incidence in hospitals for the mentally subnormal. The risks from tattooing were emphasized by an outbreak with 34 cases reported in 1979 in the South of England (Limentani *et al.*, 1979), and eventually led to the writing of a code of practice for tattoo artists.

There were of course considerable developments in diagnostic methods for hepatitis virus infection, and workers in the Virus Reference Laboratory studied both IgG and IgM antibodies to the surface, core and e antigens. The Standards Laboratory continued to evaluate diagnostic kits and new methods. A marmoset colony was established at Colindale and was successful in breeding the animals and in the production of hepatitis virus A antigen.

Reviewing "infective jaundice" as a whole in 1970, the Chief Medical Officer commented that the great majority of cases occur in the community and to a large extent among children, and this has continued to be the pattern; they had been diagnosed by exclusion as hepatitis A virus (HAV) infections, and it was not until the late 1970s that a routine laboratory diagnostic test for HAV became available (Mortimer *et al.*, 1979). These new methods were used in the study of an outbreak of hepatitis A attributable to the consumption of mussels imported from Ireland in 1978, and also for the dramatic outbreak due, surprisingly, to the consumption of frozen raspberries at a dinner at the Society of Apothecaries in 1980.

In addition to hepatitis A and B there remain a number of cases of "non-A, non-B" (NANB) hepatitis; Craske, working first at Poole and later at Manchester, recognized such cases among patients with haemophilia and other disorders requiring repeated transfusions of blood and blood products (Craske *et al.*, 1978).

Smallpox

The decade 1970–80 saw smallpox's final fling, in two incidents, both redounding to the discredit of laboratories. In 1973 a technician working at the London School of Hygiene and Tropical Medicine became infected in a laboratory and before the disease was diagnosed had infected two visitors to the hospital in which she was nursed; both later died. This naturally produced a vigorous and critical response and the DHSS set up an official tribunal of inquiry, chaired by Mr P.J. Cox, QC, the report of which contained many far-reaching proposals, referred to already (pp. 135 and 140).

In 1978 a technician in the Birmingham University Medical School contracted smallpox and, although the mechanism of transfer was obscure, she must have been infected from the virological laboratory in the same building. The surveillance of the numerous contacts was greatly assisted by the Communicable Disease Surveillance Centre, which had been set up following the recommendations of the inquiry into the previous outbreak.

In 1979 the World Health Organization finally declared smallpox eradicated from the world.

Antibiotics

Research on antibiotics has never been particularly prominent among PHLS activities, perhaps because there has not often been the need to seek research grants from drug manufacturers. However, the value of metronidazole in the treatment and prophylaxis of infection after bowel surgery was first recognized in the Newcastle and Luton PHLS laboratories and the latter, particularly, conducted a long series of clinical trials (Luton and Dunstable Hospital, 1974, 1975).

Antibiotic susceptibility testing has necessarily been a routine activity of all the laboratories; Brown, working first from Colindale and later at Cambridge, demonstrated some of the defects in the paper discs used by most workers. The part played by the Tuberculosis Reference Laboratory in improving standards of antibiotic susceptibility testing of tubercle bacilli has already been noted. The Cross-Infection, Salmonella, Enteric and Venereal Diseases Reference Laboratories all had programmes to measure the prevalence of resistant strains. The Enteric Reference Laboratory's studies (and those of the Division of Enteric Pathogens) have in many cases included analysis of the R-factors and the plasmids mediating the resistance.

Gastro-intestinal cancer

In the Bacterial Metabolism Research Laboratory, Dr M.J. Hill and his colleagues continued work on two principal research themes, both concerned with the possible role of bacteria in carcinogenesis, that we had initiated when we were working together at St Mary's Hospital Medical School. It was postulated that bacteria in the large bowel might convert bile acids to carcinogens, and the idea was attractive in that it could be reconciled with the epidemiological evidence that colon cancer is in some way related to fat intake, which increases bile secretion. In pursuit of this idea, the laboratory carried out a large prospective study in which faecal samples were collected from some 8000 volunteers to see whether either bile acid concentration or bacterial content could predict large-bowel cancer. Studies were also made of patients with chronic ulcerative colitis, who have a high risk of developing cancer. There is some evidence that a particular group of clostridia, which can dehydrogenate the steroid nucleus, may well be important.

The second theme has been the study of the possible involvement of bacteria in producing nitrosamines from nitrates, and a putative connection with stomach cancer. Both these projects are long-term, and have been supported by funds from the Cancer Research Campaign and the Department of the Environment.

The Centre for Applied Microbiology and Research

The Ministry of Defence (and its predecessor departments) had run a microbiological research laboratory at Porton Down in Wiltshire since the early days of the 1939–45 war, when it was concerned with investigating the possibilities of bacterial warfare. After the war ended the laboratory developed, largely under the leadership of D.W. Henderson, into a substantial microbiological research institute, interested in the mechanisms of airborne infection and of the pathogenesis of bacterial and viral infections. From 1956 it was known as the Microbiological Research Establishment (MRE). During the late 1960s and 1970s there was great pressure from the Ministry to reduce the size of the establishment, and for it to attract work for which it could be paid. In this it achieved some success, but by about 1975 the Ministry had decided that it could no longer agree to indefinite support for MRE. The Central Policy Review Staff (the "Think Tank") and later the Medical Research Council set up reviews of the establishment's activities and long-term potential, the eventual outcome of which was, in January 1978, an invitation from the Government to the PHLS Board to accept management responsibility for a civil institute to be derived from, and using the buildings and equipment of, the MRE.

The Board, while recognizing that it would be difficult, if not impossible, to refuse this "invitation", saw advantages and disadvantages for the PHLS. On the one hand there were at Porton some activities very relevant to a national public health laboratory service: the secure laboratories for research on and diagnosis of very dangerous pathogens (such as Lassa and Ebola viruses), experience in vaccine development and small-scale production, and the long-standing interest in microbial pathogenicity, laboratory safety and airborne infection. On the other hand, the Board was sensitive to associating the Service with an institution that had, under the Ministry of Defence, been concerned with secret work and protection against bacterial warfare. And there were several activities proposed for the new laboratory that were outside the Service's existing interests: the manufacture of various bacterial enzymes and the extraction of hormone from pituitary glands, as well as the newly developing field of biotechnology and genetic engineering. The Board's eventual acceptance of the Secretary of State's invitation was therefore hedged about with a substantial list of conditions, although it had to be satisfied with a response from the Secretary of State that he would give the Board general support and funds to enable it to develop the new centre without prejudice to the development of the existing PHLS. The Secretary of State also expressed the hope, however, that the Board would develop income-generating activities in the new centre, that could in part offset its costs.

Through the second half of 1977 and all of 1978 there were extensive discussions on the structure of the new centre, its work programme and staffing, and its name, a major element in all of these being a desire to create what would be seen as a new institute, integrated with the existing PHLS, utilizing the skills and expertise of the old, and not simply a change of name and administration. An important part of this policy was the insistence by the Board that the staff of the new institute should be appointed afresh, even if they had been on the staff of MRE, and on terms and conditions of service appropriate to the rest of the PHLS. After prolonged negotiations with the representatives of the staff, these points were conceded, and the posts on the staff of the new Centre for Applied Microbiology and Research were advertised and filled on the advice of appropriate selection committees. The PHLS Act, giving the Secretary of State for Social Services the power to include the activities of the new centre in the terms of reference of the PHLS Board, became law on 29 March 1979, and the Centre started to operate on 1 April 1979. An account of the development of the Centre, and its relation to the rest of the PHLS, as well as the effect of the grafting into it of the new Centre, will have to await a time when the perspectives are clearer, and are not discussed in this essay.

Public Health Laboratory Services in Europe

The preceding chapters have recorded the development of the public health laboratory services in England and Wales, with a brief sketch of the situation during the first three decades of the century and a more detailed account of the evolution of the national services that grew from the war-time emergency organization. Before attempting a final summary of the work of the PHLS it may be of some interest to note some of the ways in which services with the same broad objectives have developed in other countries in Europe. In 1976 the PHLS organized the first of a series of meetings of the Heads of Public Health Microbiological Services in Europe and one of the items on the agenda of the first meeting was a review of these services; for this meeting the European Office of the World Health Organization had prepared a summary paper, from which the information presented here is largely drawn.

During the 1880s and subsequently a number of countries established large central institutes for public health, in some cases supported by district laboratories. After 1918 there was more emphasis on decentralization, and later the development of tiered systems with regional and area laboratories of one form or another.

Most countries now have some form of central institute for epidemiology and public health microbiology; countries with a federal system of government (Germany, Austria, Switzerland, Yugoslavia) have several institutes in the different provinces of the federation. These central institutes ordinarily provide reference services, similar to those provided by the PHLS central laboratory at Colindale, and many of them organize the external quality assessment schemes for their countries. In the Netherlands the central laboratory has had a policy of contracting out some of its reference services to university or other specialist laboratories. Many of the central institutes have laboratories for chemical and physical examinations in support of the community public health services.

The relation of the central institute to peripheral laboratories varies. In the Scandinavian countries the institute is responsible for guiding and co-ordinating the work of the laboratories, situated in hospitals or university departments, that provide the public health microbiology services for the community. These laboratories commonly also serve as clinical microbiology laboratories for hospitals. Similarly, in the eastern European countries the central institutes are generally responsible for guiding the peripheral laboratories ("sanitary/epidemiological stations") that provide the epidemiological and public health microbiological services, but they are not directly concerned with the administration of the entirely separate clinical laboratories in hospitals. In France, Germany, Italy and Belgium the central institutes have no formal links with the peripheral laboratories apart from the provision of reference services and quality assessment.

The pattern of "area" laboratories also varies greatly. In Scandinavia the public health microbiology is generally provided by the laboratories in hospitals or universities, the latter associated with hospitals. In the eastern European countries (the Soviet Union, Czechoslovakia, Hungary, Rumania, Bulgaria) there are networks of national or provincial sanitary/epidemiological stations, quite separate from the laboratories serving the hospitals. These laboratories may be responsible for chemical analyses as well as microbiological.

In several countries (e.g. France, Germany, Italy and Belgium) the peripheral services are provided by a variety of laboratories, in universities or hospitals, private profit-making laboratories, or municipal public health laboratories. Again these laboratories may carry out chemical investigations as well as microbiological.

In Scotland, as noted earlier, the university departments have continued to provide the public health microbiology services, supplemented in some areas by hospital laboratories and in Glasgow by a municipal public health laboratory. Scotland has no central institute although it has a tuberculosis reference laboratory; central epidemiological services are provided by the Communicable Diseases (Scotland) Unit, which is one of the Common Services Units of the National Health Service.

Forty Years of Microbiology for the Public Health

The demands that the Public Health puts on a microbiological service, in respect of infective diseases, can perhaps be subsumed under five headings: identification of infections in individuals and advice on management; collation and distribution of the reports of these infections so as to detect patterns of outbreaks or epidemics; research into methods for identification or control; generation of advice on national public health policies; and education, both professional and lay. By way of final synthesis, it may be of interest to look at the 40 years' contribution of the EPHLS and PHLS in these terms.

Laboratory tests to answer the question "Is this person's illness attributable to infection and if so how should it be treated?" constitute the microbiologists' bread and butter, and by 1980 PHLS laboratories were probably doing some 5 million of these tests annually, this constituting perhaps 15 per cent of all such tests done in England and Wales.

The 40 years' evolution of the PHLS from a service primarily providing diagnostic facilities for medical officers of health and general practitioners, and concerned with

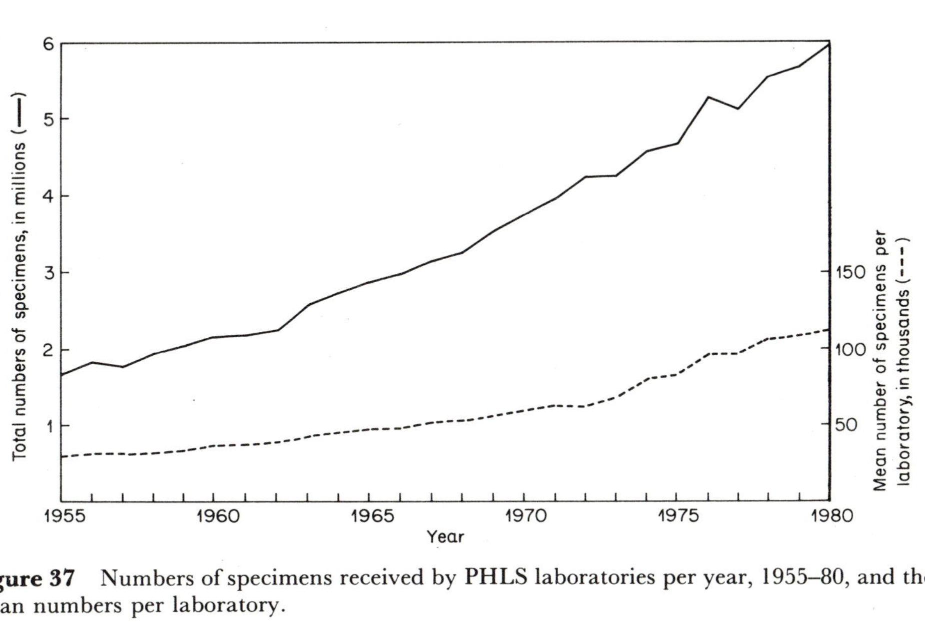

Figure 37 Numbers of specimens received by PHLS laboratories per year, 1955–80, and the mean numbers per laboratory.

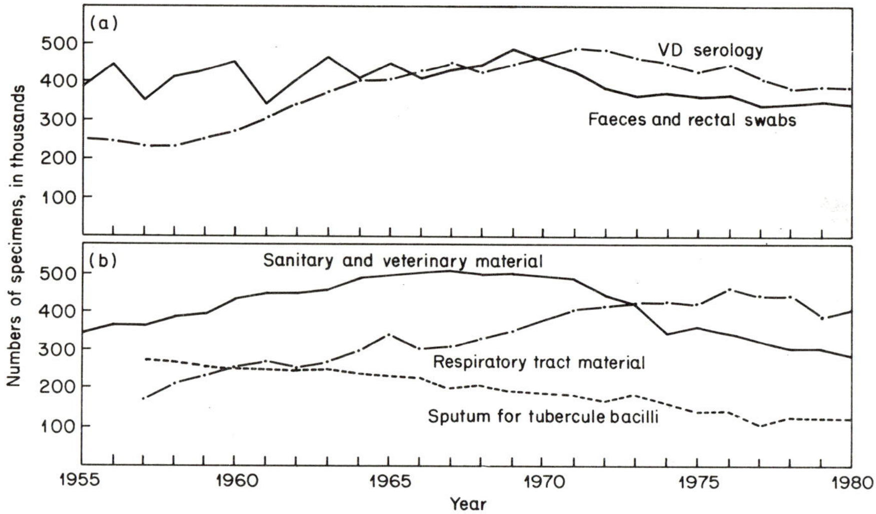

Figure 38 Numbers of specimens received for examination for specific types of examination, 1955–80: (a) specimens for VD serology (— · —) and faeces and rectal swabs for bacteriological examination (———); (b) respiratory tract material (— · —), sputum for tubercule bacilli (-----) and sanitary and veterinary material (———).

infections in the community, to one seeing public health as intimately concerned with all aspects of infective disease, in hospital and in the community, is well illustrated by the changes in the nature of the tests being carried out, as illustrated in the "workload" statistics displayed in Figures 37–41. Few figures are available for the years prior to 1955, but from then on the numbers of specimens received by the laboratories have been collected in a reasonably consistent form.

The total number of specimens rose inexorably, increasing fourfold in the 25 years to 1980 (Figure 37), and this increase was only to a small extent accounted for by changes in the number of laboratories. The overall rise is a compound of decline in the numbers in a few specimen categories and little change over the years in a few (Figure 38), and dramatic expansion in three (Figure 39). In 1957, 20 per cent of the specimens were faeces or rectal swabs, and 20 per cent "sanitary" – food, milk, water and veterinary. Of the 446,000 respiratory tract specimens, 62 per cent were for the examination for tubercle bacilli (and incidentally about 23 per cent of these were examined only by direct microscopy). The number of faecal specimens fluctuated considerably from year to year, and after about 1969 showed a slight but steady decline; as a percentage of the total workload, however, faecal specimens declined from 20 per cent to about 6 per cent. Similarly, the sanitary specimens, after increasing in numbers until around 1968, declined steadily, and the corresponding figures were 20 per cent for 1955 and 5 per cent for 1980. Serum specimens for the diagnosis of venereal disease increased steadily from 1955 to 1971 (from 250,000 to 492,000 per year) and then declined to about 393,000, or 7 per cent of the workload. These categories of specimens are all those that could be regarded as of community public health interest (despite the arguments early

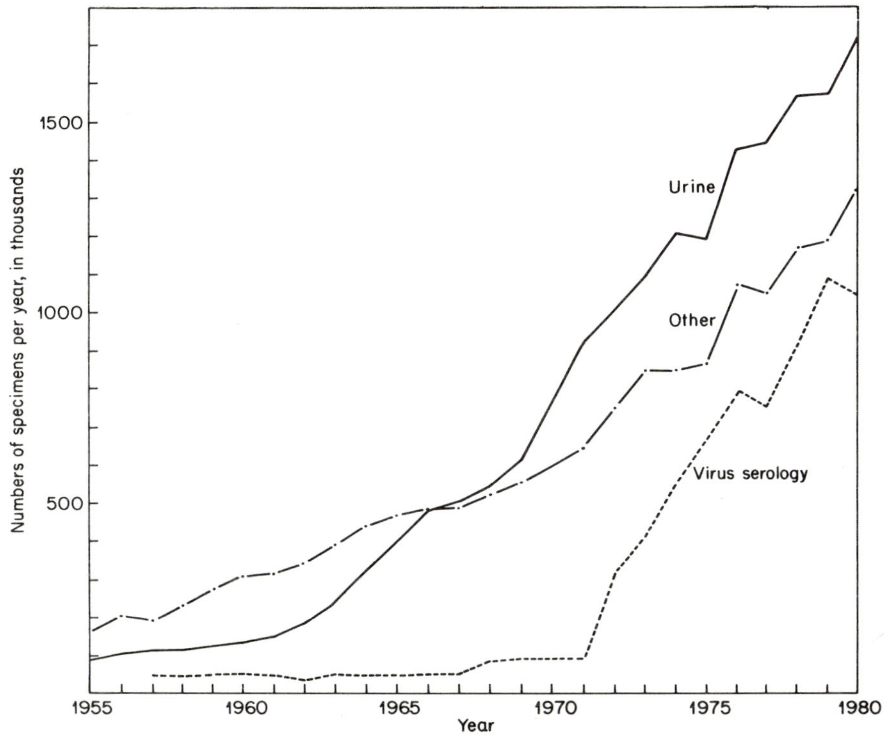

Figure 39 Numbers of specimens received for urine bacteriology (———), for bacteriology of specimens other than urine, respiratory tract material and faeces (— · —) and for virus serology, including toxoplasma and chlamydia (-----), 1955–80.

in the 1950s that tuberculosis and venereal disease work should properly fall to the hospital service – p. 55).

Three categories of specimens largely account for the increase in the totals (Figure 39). Two of these certainly reflect the developing responsibilities for hospital bacteriology, namely urines and "other human", representing blood cultures, "pus" swabs, antibiotic susceptibility tests and so forth. Both categories increased in numbers steeply through the whole period and by 1980 together accounted for 51 per cent of the total specimen numbers. The third category to show a great increase was "virus serology", reflecting the development of tests for the hepatitis surface antigen (HBsAg) and the call to determine the rubella antibody status of pregnant women and adult candidates for vaccination.

The outstanding diagnostic developments of the four decades to 1980 have been in virology. No longer is it legitimate to assert that "it must be a virus" as the cause of some malady in which no bacterial pathogen can be detected: if it is a virus there is a good chance that it can be demonstrated. By 1980, PHLS laboratories, all but 10 of which carried out diagnostic virology, received some 166,000 specimens for virus isolation or detection by electron microscopy (Figure 40). Although this represents less

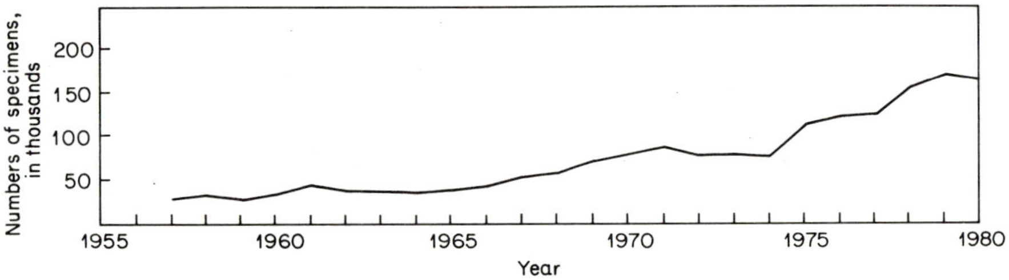

Figure 40 Numbers of specimens received for isolation of viruses or detection by electron microscopy, 1955–80.

than 3 per cent of the total specimen numbers, the proportion of time and material dedicated to their examination must constitute far more than 3 per cent.

It needs to be stressed that the involvement in clinical microbiology for hospitals has been seen as an essential ingredient for a service that has the function of monitoring and advising on all aspects of the public health as it concerns infective diseases: a great proportion of the patients with infections are to be found in general hospitals. And general practitioners having the care of patients in their homes now use the laboratory services of general hospitals to provide them with diagnostic assistance. In any case, as we have seen, infections can and do spread within the hospitals themselves.

The methods for carrying out diagnostic tests have been a continuing topic of research and development that generated no fewer than 800 papers and other publications between 1940 and 1980, and even this does not reflect the whole: there can hardly ever have been a meeting of the Staff Committee or a Director's Meeting without some formal or informal report of a technical development.

The PHLS has traditionally rejected the idea of insisting that all laboratories should use one standard method (except where this is statutorily required), believing in the value of diversity and initiative. It is, however, an unfortunate corrollary to this that some may stick to methods that are not the most effective or not the most economical. One of the prime objectives of the regular meetings of PHLS directors has been to provide opportunities for all to hear of improvements (or fallacies) in accepted or new methods. Moreover, the organization of the "quality assessment" scheme, which the PHLS has provided for the whole of the United Kingdom, is a broadly based attempt to improve laboratory diagnosis, by revealing to its practitioners where they fail. By 1981 some 100 specimens were being issued each year to over 500 laboratories. This must in time lead to a better service, though it has to be admitted that it is difficult to devise a scheme that penetrates very deeply into the diagnostic process, and even more difficult to construct one that tests the quality of interpretation.

The detailed characterization of the microbes isolated in the diagnostic tests, while not necessarily important for the management of the individual patient, is often essential for studies of epidemiology. This characterization may be taxonomic, and the National Collection of Type Cultures (NCTC) has had an active programme of research into methods for distinguishing valid taxa, as well as into the vexatious territory of nomenclature. Of course, by the period of this review, most of the major taxa of pathogenic organisms had been delineated, and new work in this field has mostly been in the direction of picking out relevant groups from the morass of "also rans". The NCTC has provided a diagnostic service for many of these "difficult" groups of bacteria.

For the more common pathogenic bacteria and viruses, epidemiological inquiry generally demands a finer characterization: type identification. This has been the primary function of the reference laboratories, already part of the Service during the war years. Originally most type identification relied on serological identification of type antigens, but the life-span of the EPHLS and PHLS has seen the development of a range of typing methods other than serological. Phage typing was developed by Felix for *Salmonella typhi* in the 1940s, as was phage typing for *Staphylococcus aureus*, by Wilson and Atkinson. The Enteric Reference Laboratory, which had applied phage typing methods with great profit to *S. typhimurium* and a few other salmonella serotypes, led the way when further refinement was possible with the methods of molecular biology that could be applied to the typing of the factors responsible for resistance to antibiotics. Quite recently similar methods have been used to determine the geographical origin of strains of penicillinase-producing gonococci.

These are but examples; the 40 years have seen more than 450 publications on taxonomy and type identification, the great proportion emanating from the reference laboratories, one of whose main functions has been research into the recognition of new types, and the validation of new types defined by others (often with an accepted international responsibility).

However, the primary function of the reference laboratories has been to support the first-line diagnostic laboratories in the PHLS and in the hospital service by identifying or typing strains of microbes to help in the investigation into the origins of infections, or examining sera for specific antibodies. The Annual Report for 1979 reveals that, in that year, some 52,000 strains of bacteria, viruses, fungi and mycoplasmas were examined in the reference laboratories, together with some 34,000 sera. In addition, reference experts in peripheral laboratories also provided typing services (Table 3), though the number of strains examined is not recorded.

The bacteria that are received by the reference laboratories but cannot be identified constitute the stimulus to much of their research work, especially when the relation between the reference laboratory and the peripheral laboratory sending the strains is such that the reference laboratory knows that there is a genuine epidemiological or clinical need for further tests. There can be no doubt that, over the period of the last 40 years, the reference laboratories have benefited greatly from the ready interactive relations with the peripheral PHLS laboratories and with some epidemiologically active hospital laboratories in developing and refining the typing methods and defining their significance. Although there are now university departments of microbiology that offer identification services on a limited scale for organisms in which they have a particular interest, the typing services developed and provided by the PHLS have been a contribution to the public health of quite outstanding importance.

Much of the work of the first-line diagnostic laboratories and of the subsequent type identification requires the production of high quality reagents, particularly antisera and antigens. The PHLS Standards Laboratory, now part of the Division of Microbiological Reagents and Quality Control (DMRQC), has built up an enviable reputation for the range and quality of the reagents it produces, and for a long while it was virtually the only British source for many of the reagents used in virological diagnosis. In this field, as well as in the bacterial, there are now also high-quality commercial suppliers, and the activity of DMRQC may be expected to move towards the quality control of these reagents.

It is normal practice for laboratories to keep records of their isolations of specific pathogens to detect undue prevalence of infection, which may indicate a local "outbreak" or some lapse in aseptic precautions. The special contribution of the PHLS has been to create systems for carrying out this surveillance on a national scale. This is achieved both through the routine activities of the reference laboratories, and through the weekly reporting, by PHLS and hospital laboratories, first to the Epidemiological Research Laboratory and since 1977 to the Communicable Disease Surveillance Centre. The Weekly Summary of reports initiated by Wilson in the early EPHLS days has developed and grown into the current *Communicable Disease Report*. These systems – reference laboratory observations and weekly reports – have on many occasions led to the recognition of widespread epidemics. For example, the periodic nation-wide prevalence of mycoplasma infections, and the cyclical character of the central nervous system infections due to echoviruses and other viruses would not otherwise have been detected. In the fields of food poisoning the national collection of reports has on occasion revealed that a number of separate outbreaks had in fact a common source, such as a food manufacturer, importer or distributor. On other occasions it has been instrumental in recognizing the dangers from some new foodstuff, as in the case of Chinese frozen egg, or medicament, exemplified by the "epidemic" of salmonellosis in children treated with pancreatin. The discovery of some of these sources has been responsible for the subsequent introduction of new hygiene regulations, such as those requiring pasteurization of egg products, the control of protein in animal feeds, or the insistence on the use of chlorinated water for cooling canned meat and vegetables during manufacture.

The recognition of an outbreak of infection – whether by observation of an undue prevalence of some particular microbe in specimens examined in the laboratory, or by clinical reports – commonly calls for further laboratory and epidemiological work. This is what the EPHLS and PHLS were constituted to do, at a time when facilities for such work were quite inadequate in the fragmented hospital service. Notwithstanding the growing workload from the acute hospital bacteriology, investigation of small and large outbreaks has continued to be an important element in PHLS work, and the traditional epidemiological activities of the central and peripheral laboratory directors have been greatly assisted in the last few years by the epidemiologists on the staff of the Communicable Disease Surveillance Centre and the Epidemiological Research Laboratory. About 200 of these investigations have led to publication in medical journals and many others have been summarized more briefly in the Weekly Summary or the *Communicable Disease Report*. In the three years 1977–9, a total of 95 investigations by PHLS laboratories of outbreaks of infections were reported in the *Communicable Disease Report*: 65 were gastro-intestinal infections in hospital or community, 15 virus infections and 18 other bacterial infections. More general epidemiological studies, based on a series of outbreaks, or on wider studies, have been reported in nearly 500 publications.

The data generated by the regular reporting of laboratory results does not, of course, always lead to action, even when it demonstrates the existence of a widespread epidemic, for we still have no way of controlling many of the infections we can diagnose. The accumulation of more and more precise knowledge of these infections may be thought of as something of a luxury, but is surely a luxury that an advanced country ought to enjoy, for it is only by accumulating such knowledge that one can judge whether specific control measures are needed, or theoretically feasible.

Over the years PHLS laboratories and epidemiologists have made numerous studies to explore methods for the control of infection. Within months of its mobilization, the EPHLS was investigating the control of outbreaks of diphtheria. Innumerable studies have been made of the control of food poisoning and diarrhoeal diseases. The work in renal dialysis units was strikingly successful in controlling hepatitis. Many studies were made of methods for the control of other hospital-acquired infections, and some of them led to new policies for aspects of hospital design and practice, though it cannot be said that many were unequivocally shown to have as clear an effect as the work on preventing hepatitis in dialysis units. The study of the frequency of complications following measles served as an important stimulus to government to introduce general measles vaccination; the whooping cough work demonstrated the initial success, the later partial failure, and the subsequent improvement of that vaccination campaign.

The national vaccination policies and the various hygiene regulations commonly call for laboratory as well as epidemiological monitoring. PHLS surveillance of the poliomyelitis, measles, whooping cough and BCG programmes has been mentioned, and a substantial amount of the area laboratories' work on sanitary specimens consists of routine examinations to check that standards are being met. Overall, this latter activity has declined over the years, with the eradication of bovine tuberculosis and the near eradication of brucellosis, as well as the setting up of their own laboratories by the new large water authorities. It has never been United Kingdom policy to rely heavily on routine microbiological tests for food hygiene. The fact that PHLS laboratories perform the tests required for the control of food and drink, as well as the routine public health microbiology for the investigation of infective illness, ensures that the medical relevance (or irrelevance) of the sanitary bacteriology can be kept in mind. Furthermore, it is a great advantage that there is no financial incentive to the proliferation of tests on foodstuffs, or on food handlers.

Lastly, education and training. From 1945 new recruits to the PHLS have always had an organized training programme, involving a rotation between laboratories and an academic year to study for the Diploma in Bacteriology, or latterly an MSc in Medical Microbiology. The training programme was also ideally suited for those aiming for membership of the Royal College of Pathologists, as virtually all medically qualified trainees now do. The PHLS has also encouraged members of staff to attend other specialized training courses, and has funded them to do so.

What is more, ever since the end of the war the Central Public Health Laboratory has been a magnet for visitors from all parts of Britain and indeed all over the world. The laboratory has never, in the past, had adequate space to run training courses for more than two or three persons, but there can hardly ever have been a week in any of the 35 years when there were not several short- or long-stay visitors in one or other of the reference laboratories. Many have been sponsored by the World Health Organization, others by their own governments. The exchange has not been all one way; many of the visitors staying for longer periods have made active contributions to the research activities of the departments, and many of those trained in particular techniques, especially type identification, have continued as collaborators in international studies on their return home. Educational activities have by no means been confined to the Central Public Health Laboratory; the Leeds and Bath laboratories have been particularly active in courses for environmental health officers, but the staff of virtually all laboratories contribute in one way or another. The PHLS has also run a number of short courses in London for the British Council, aimed at public health workers from overseas. Members of the staff have contributed to numberless courses and seminars run by universities and professional bodies, and many have also travelled abroad at the request of the World Health Organization, the British Council, overseas governments and others to advise on services and to train personnel.

A substantial part of the Public Health's need for acute microbiological assistance is provided by the 350 or so National Health Service hospital laboratories, some of which also do a limited amount of sanitary bacteriology and a few, particularly those in the universities, provide limited reference services. The PHLS has, in recent years, been carrying out perhaps 15 per cent of the acute diagnostic bacteriology, and a much larger proportion of the acute diagnostic virology, thus providing an invaluable and accessible sample of the infections prevalent in the country. The consultants in hospital laboratories are certainly more epidemiologically oriented than their predecessors of 40, or even 30, years ago and there is no longer the discrepancy in standards of microbiological practice that certainly existed in the early days between PHLS and many hospital laboratories. The chief advantages seen for retaining a system in which some 50 of the country's clinical laboratories are designated as having specific public health functions are that it provides for a more systematic sampling frame for observing the pattern of infective disease, that it makes possible a rapid, co-ordinated response to calls for specific information on "new" infections or new trends in old, and that it provides the community public health services with a network of laboratories trained in and committed to the support of the control of infection.

The more nearly unique contributions of the PHLS have been in the reference services and in epidemiology, the latter growing in importance over the years as the need for laboratory-based epidemiology has increased and the medical officers of health were succeeded by community physicians with many roles other than the control of infectious disease. The reference services and the analytical aspects of the epidemiological work have been largely centralized at Colindale, but their development as resources available to the whole country has certainly been made possible by their close relations within one national Service with the regional and area laboratories, a Service realizing the aims that Topley defined in 1938, and that was created to such a large extent by the vision and skill of G.S. Wilson.

Appendix

The tables and figures that appear on the following pages supplement the information given earlier in the text as regards the various laboratories of the PHLS (constituent, associated and recognized) during its development. Information is also provided with regard to members of the PHLS Boards, finance, staffing, and other items of interest.

Appendix Table 1 Constituent area and regional laboratories of the EPHLS and PHLS, 1939–80
[O, opened; C, closed; (N), new construction; (C), conversion; R, regional (by 1980)]

Laboratory	Date	Address	Director	Additional remarks
Aberystwyth	O: 1939	Dairy Research Institute	A. C. Jones	
	1943	Cardiganshire General Hospital	M. V. N. Sudds	
	C: 1961			After an interval, continued as a sub-laboratory to Carmarthen till 1965
Barnard Castle	O: 1939	Barnard Castle School	S. H. Warren	Run from Durham University
	C: 1941			
Bath	O: 1952	Manor Hospital (C)	P. G. Mann	J. Mackey locum director 1966–7
Bedford	O: 1951	General Hospital (N)	W. F. Lane	
	C: 1973			
Birkenhead	O: 1948	Municipal Laboratory, Hamilton Square	J. M. Ritchie	
	1959		J. D. Abbott	
	C: 1960			Transferred to Chester
Birmingham, R	O: 1950	City Laboratory, Great Charles Street	B. R. Sandiford	
	1965		J. G. P. Hutchinson	
	1969	East Birmingham Hospital (N)		Integrated with hospital laboratory, and close association with Regional Virus Laboratory (T. H. Flewett)
Bradford	O: 1947	City Laboratory, Edmund Street	A. J. H. Tomlinson	
	1953		H. G. M. Smith	
	C: 1973			
Brighton	O: 1949	Royal Sussex County Hospital (N)	J. E. Jameson	
	1951	Same, new laboratory		
	1973		B. Thom	
Bristol, R	O: 1959	University Bacteriology Laboratory, Canynge Hall	H. R. Cayton	
	1969	Myrtle Road (N)		
	1978		A. E. Jephcott	
Cambridge, R	O: 1939	University School of Pathology, Tennis Court Road	F. Griffith	
	1940		A. W. Downie	

		1943		E. T. C. Spooner	
		1944		A. M. McFarlan (acting)	
		1946		R. M. Fry	
		1950	New laboratory, same address (N)		
		1963		G. R. E. Naylor	
		1973	New Addenbrookes Hospital (N)		
		1976		C. E. D. Taylor	
Canterbury	O:	1939	Kings School	A. M. McFarlan	
	C:	1939			
Cardiff, R	O:	1939	Institute of Preventive Medicine	V. D. Allison	
		1946		G. J. G. King	
		1947		S. Thomson	
		1948			Cardiff and County Laboratory absorbed
		1951	Additional laboratory, Royal Infirmary		
		1970		C. H. L. Howells	
		1971	University Hospital of Wales, The Heath (retaining Royal Infirmary)		
		1977			Took over work of Newport PHL
Carlisle	O:	1955	Cumberland Infirmary	D. G. Davies	
Carmarthen	O:	1940	Penlan Road	R. M. Fry	
		1946		M. T. Parker	
		1948		W. Kwantes	
		1956		M. H. Hughes	
		1958		H. D. S. Morgan	
		1961	West Wales General Hospital (N)		
Chelmsford	O:	1956	Chelmsford and Essex Hospital (N)	R. Pilsworth	
		1974			Took over work of Southend PHL
Chester	O:	1960	Chester City Hospital (N)	P. M. Poole	Took over work of Birkenhead PHL Sub-laboratory at Wrexham Hospital (D. C. J. Bassett), 1963–5
Cirencester	O:	1948	Practice offices	R. E. Hope Simpson	Epidemiological work in association with general practice
		1960	Dyer Street, small laboratory and office		
	C:	1973			

Appendix Table 1 *(contd)*

Laboratory	Date	Address	Director	Additional remarks
Colchester	O: 1939		P. H. Martin	
	C: 1940			Transferred to Ipswich
Conway/Rhyl	O: 1939	Fisheries Experimental Station	D. T. Robinson	Originally sub-laboratory to Liverpool
	1943		E. D. Hoare	
	1946		A. J. Kingsley Smith	
	1948	Bryn Hyfryd, converted house		
	1961			Senior bacteriologist to Rhyl Hospital
	1966		F. B. Jackson	
	1980	Ysbyty Glan Clwyd, Bodelwyddan (N)		
Coventry	O: 1949	Coventry and Warwick Hospital (C)	R. E. Jones	
	1958		P. M. Poole (acting)	
			J. E. M. Whitehead	
	1973	Same address, new laboratory (N)	E. M. Finnie (*d.* 1975)	
	1976		P. R. Mortimer	
Derby	O: 1958	Derbyshire Royal Infirmary (N)	J. L. G. Iredale	
	1965		B. W. Barton	
	1975		R. Darnell (acting)	
	C: 1977			
Dorchester	O: 1951	County Laboratory, Glyde Path Road	G. H. Tee	
	1979		P. Gill	Sub-laboratory at Herrison Hospital for virus work
Epsom	O: 1946	West Hill House (C)	D. M. Stone	
	1961		D. R. Gamble	
	1964	West Park Hospital (C)		
Exeter	O: 1940	County Laboratory, Dix's Field	E. P. Hicks	
	1941		J. G. Cruickshank	
	1945		B. Moore	
	1959	Gandy Street (grounds of old university buildings) (C)		
	1966	Royal Devon and Exeter Hospital (N)		
	1977		R. J. C. Hart	

Gloucester	O:	1939	County Mental Hospital	R. M. Fry	
	C:	1940			
	O:	1964	Gloucester Royal Hospital	A. E. Wright	
		1979		A. P. C. H. Roome (acting)	
Guildford	O:	1953	St Luke's Hospital	G. T. Cook	
		1967	Same address, new laboratory (N)		
		1971		J. R. Davies	
		1977		R. Y. Cartwright	
Harrogate	O:	1951	Harrogate and District General Hospital	L. A. Little	
		1954			Northallerton PHL in charge
	C:	1956			
Hereford	O:	1942	County Laboratory	R. E. Jones	
		1949		W. H. J. Baker (acting)	
		1950		D. R. Christie	
		1951	County Hospital, Hereford (C)		
		1974	Same address, new laboratory (N)		
Holt	O:	1939	Gresham's School	A. Q. Wells	
	C:	1939			
Horsham	O:	1939	Christ's Hospital School	J. G. Cruickshank	
		1941		L. Foulds	
	C:	1945			
Hull	O:	1948	County Analyst's Laboratory, High Street	C. L. Greening	
		1952		J. H. McCoy	
		1967	Royal Infirmary (N)		
		1980		S. L. Mawer	
Ipswich	O:	1940	County Laboratory, Bond Street	P. H. Martin	
		1949	Borough General Hospital (N)		
		1959		J. M. S. Dixon	
		1966		P. K. Fraser	
		1975	Same address, new laboratory (N)		
		1976		J. V. T. Gostling	
Kirkby Lonsdale	O:	1939	Grammar School	J. W. Orr	Run from Leeds University
	C:	1939			
Leeds, R	O:	1955	Seacroft Hospital (N)	G. B. Ludlam	
		1972		G. L. Gibson	

Appendix Table 1 (*contd*)

Laboratory	Date	Address	Director	Additional remarks
Leicester	O: 1940	Isolation Hospital, Groby Road (C)	R. Knox	
	1945		B. P. Marmion (acting)	
	1946		E. H. Gillespie	
	1952		N. S. Mair	
	1978		C. J. Mitchell	
	1980	Royal Infirmary (N)		
Lincoln	O: 1939	Technical College	J. M. Croll	
	1947	St Edmunds Chambers, Bank Street (C)		
	1950	County Hospital (N)		
	1971		J. G. Wallace	
Liverpool, R	O: 1955	City Bacteriological Laboratory, Mount Pleasant	D. T. Robinson	
	1956			University department left laboratory
	1965		G. C. Turner	
	1972	Fazakerley Hospital (N)		
London				
Camberwell	O: 1948	Camberwell Research Laboratory, Denmark Hill	G. Bousfield	
	C: 1953			
Central Middlesex	O: 1968	Central Middlesex Hospital, new hospital laboratory	C. E. D. Taylor	
	1970	Same address, temporary laboratory		
	1974	Same address, new laboratory (N)		
	1976		D. A. McSwiggan	
County Hall	O: 1953	County Hall, Westminster (C)	A. J. H. Tomlinson	Took over work of Camberwell
	1968		J. R. Davies	
	1972		C. Dulake	
	C: 1973			Transferred to Dulwich
Dulwich	O: 1973	Dulwich Hospital (N)	C. Dulake	Transferred from County Hall
Hither Green	O: 1949	Park Hospital, Southern Group Laboratory	J. E. McCartney	

		1952		E. H. Bailey (acting)	
	C:	1953			
London School of Hygiene	O:	1940	London School of Hygiene and Tropical Medicine	W. M. Scott	
	C:	1941			
Tooting	O:	1966	St George's Hospital, Tooting (C)	D. G. Fleck	
Whipps Cross	O:	1970	Whipps Cross Hospital (C)	B. Thom	
		1974		B. Chattopadhyay	
Luton	O:	1947	Municipal Laboratory, Town Hall	J. A. Pitt Evans	
		1949		J. H. C. Walker	
		1954	Luton and Dunstable Hospital (N)		
		1955		H. D. Holt	
		1967		A. T. Willis	
Maidstone	O:	1948	County Laboratory, County Hall	J. H. C. Walker	
		1956	Preston Hall (N)		
		1960		A. L. Furniss	
Manchester, R	O:	1948	Monsall Hospital	M. T. Parker	
		1961		J. O'H. Tobin	
		1964	Withington Hospital (N)		
		1975		D. M. Jones	
Middlesbrough	O:	1951	General Hospital (C)	R. Blowers	
		1967		J. A. N. Emslie (acting)	
		1968		J. G. Wallace (acting)	
		1970		P. R. Mortimer	
		1976		E. Mackay-Ferguson	
Newcastle	O:	1947	County Laboratory, High Street, Newburn	A. I. Messer	
		1948	Newcastle General Hospital		
	O:	1947	City Laboratory, General Hospital	R. Norton	
		1948			Absorbed Newburn laboratory
	O:	1947	Durham University Medical School	S. H. Warren	
		1948	Government Buildings, Ponteland Road	R. Norton	
		1956	General Hospital, new laboratory (N)	A. I. Messer	Absorbed earlier laboratories
		1959		J. H. Hale	
		1977		J. B. Selkon	

Appendix Table 1 (*contd*)

Laboratory	Date	Address	Director	Additional remarks
Newport	O: 1948	County Laboratory, County Hall	W. Panes	
	1949		R. D. Gray	
	1957	Royal Gwent Hospital, Clythra Square (N)		
	C: 1976			
Northallerton	O: 1942	County Laboratory, County Hall	W. Goldie	
	1948		E. J. Hallinan	
	1949		D. J. H. Payne	
	1951	Friarage Hospital		
	1964		J. G. Wallace	
	C: 1971			
Northampton	O: 1941	General Hospital	P. G. H. Gell (temporarily in charge)	
	1941		L. Hoyle	
	1952	Same address, new laboratory (N)		
	C: 1973			
Norwich	O: 1943	County Laboratory, Isolation Hospital	A. Macdonald	
	1948		L. M. Dowsett	
	1954	West Norwich Hospital (N)		
	1974		W. Shepherd	
Nottingham	O: 1948	City Laboratory, Cumberland Place	G. B. Ludlam	
	1949	Goldsmith Street (C)		
	1955		E. R. Mitchell	
	1966	City Hospital (C)		
	1976		M. J. Lewis	
	1977	University Hospital (N)		
Oxford, R	O: 1939	Dunn School of Pathology	W. M. Scott	
	1940		G. S. Wilson	
	1945	Radcliffe Infirmary (N)	R. Knox	
	1949		G. T. Cook (acting)	
	1949		R. L. Vollum	
	1965		W. H. H. Jebb	

		1975		J. O'H. Tobin	
		1979	John Radcliffe Hospital (N)		
Peterborough	O:	1946	Peterborough and District Hospital	C. C. B. Gilmour	
		1956		E. A. Holden	
		1958		J. C. Kelsey	
		1960		E. J. G. Glencross	
		1968	Same address, new joint laboratory (N)		
		1972	Same address, new laboratory (N)		
		1976		R. S. Jobanputra	
Plymouth	O:	1953	South Devon and East Cornwall Hospital	C. H. Jellard	
		1969		P. D. Meers	
		1972	Same address, new laboratory (C)		
		1979		P. J. Wilkinson	
Pocklington	O:	1939	Pocklington School	J. W. Goldie	Run from Leeds University
	C:	1942			Transferred to Northallerton
Poole	O:	1948	Municipal Laboratory, Municipal Buildings	G. J. G. King	
		1951	Isolation Hospital, Gloucester Road, Bournemouth		
		1969	Poole General Hospital (N)		
		1972		W. L. Hooper	
Portsmouth, R	O:	1949	Central Laboratory, Infectious Diseases Hospital, Milton Road	K. E. A. Hughes	
		1950	St Mary's Hospital (C)		
		1964		D. J. H. Payne	
Preston	O:	1958	Royal Infirmary (N)	L. Robertson	
Reading	O:	1944	Royal Berkshire Hospital		Initially under the direction of the local medical officer of health
		1946		P. Kidd	
		1948		N. Wood	
		1951	Battle Hospital		
		1967	Royal Berkshire Hospital (N)	J. V. Dadswell	
		1978	Same address, new laboratory (N)		
Salisbury	O:	1954	General Infirmary	M. S. Pereira	
		1957		P. J. Wormald	
		1966	Odstock Hospital (C)		
		1978		S. Patrick	

Appendix Table 1 *(contd)*

Laboratory	Date	Address	Director	Additional remarks
Sheffield, R	O: 1948	City General Hospital (*ex* Municipal Laboratory)	L. Gordon Cook (acting)	
	1952		E. H. Gillespie	
	1975		B. W. Barton	
Sherborne	O: 1939		E. P. Hicks	
	C: 1940			
Shrewsbury	O: 1947	Royal Salop Infirmary	A. C. Jones	
	1971	Royal Shrewsbury Hospital (N)		
	1972		C. A. Morris	
Southampton	O: 1947	Health Centre	J. M. B. Edwards	
	1948		R. I. Hutchinson	
	1963	General Hospital (N)		
	1966		J. M. Graham	
	1975		A. M. R. Mackenzie	
	1976	Same address, new laboratory (N)	P. J. Fraser (acting)	
	1978		A. D. Pearson	
Southend	O: 1948	Borough Sanatorium (Westcliff Hospital) (N)	J. O. Oliver (acting)	
	1950		R. Pilsworth	
	1956		M. A. M. Wilson	
	1958		J. A. Rycroft	
	1970	Southend General Hospital (C)		
	C: 1974			Transferred to Chelmsford
Stamford	O: 1939	Stamford School	R. Knox	
	C: 1940			Transferred to Leicester
Stafford	O: 1947	County Laboratory, Martin Street	R. I. Hutchinson	
	1947		R. N. Phease	
	1956		E. M. Mackay-Scollay	
				A. E. Wright, locum director, 1963
	1966		W. L. Hooper	
	1969		P. Cavanagh	
	C: 1975			Transferred to Stoke-on-Trent

Stoke-on-Trent	O:	1975	Stoke General Hospital (N)	P. Cavanagh	
		1976		C. R. Knappett	
Sunderland	O:	1950	Royal Infirmary	P. B. Crone	
		1953	Havelock Hospital (C)		
	C:	1973			PHLS continued administration for the regional health authority (G. Scrimgeour, director) after 1973
Swansea	O:	1956	Isolation Hospital, Crocket Road (N)	W. Kwantes	
Taunton	O:	1946	County Hall	J. A. Boycott	Initially under the local medical officer of health
		1952	Musgrave Park Hospital (N)		
		1970		J. V. S. Pether	
Tavistock	O:	1939	Kelly College	C. H. Andrewes	
	C:	1940			Transferred to Exeter
Truro	O:	1949	Royal Cornwall Infirmary	D. R. Christie	
		1950		F. D. M. Hocking (acting)	
		1964	Same address, new laboratory (N)	G. I. Barrow	
		1979		J. C. K. Mills (acting)	
		1980		W. A. Telfer Brunton	
Wakefield	O:	1947	County Laboratory, Wood Street	J. C. Colbeck	
		1948		W. F. Lane	
		1951		H. T. Findlay	
		1954		L. A. Little	
	C:	1973			
Watford	O:	1946	Peace Memorial Hospital	B. Cadness Graves	
		1967		B. R. Eaton	Sub-laboratory at Holywell Hospital
		1971	Shrodells Hospital (N)		
Wellington	O:	1939	Wrekin College	R. E. Jones	Originally run from Birmingham University
	C:	1942			Transferred to Hereford
Winchester	O:	1939	Winchester College	J. T. Duncan	
		1945		R. D. Mackenzie	
		1946	Royal Hampshire County Hospital (N)		
		1954		H. T. Findlay	
		1958		M. H. Hughes	
	C:	1975			

Appendix Table 1 (*contd*)

Laboratory	Date	Address	Director	Additional remarks
Wolverhampton	O: 1969	New Cross Hospital (N)	C. H. L. Howells	
	1971		I. A. Harper	
Worcester	O: 1948	Royal Infirmary	P. Kidd	
	1949		R. J. Henderson	
	C: 1976			PHLS contributed subsequently (M. B. Skirrow, director)

Appendix Table 2 Emergency laboratories for public health work in the London sectors, 1939

Laboratory	Situation	Director
Brentwood[a]	Brentwood School	A. B. Rosher
Hertford	Haileybury School	A. W. Downie
Harpenden[b]	Rothamsted Experiment Station	J. M. Alston
Watford	Hospital	A. R. Berrie
Ealing	Hospital	A. B. Porteous
Northwood[c]	Merchant Taylors' School	C. J. C. Britton
Slough[a]	Industrial laboratory	G. W. Goodhart
Guildford[a]	County School	R. F. L. Hewlett
Epsom	Epsom College	T. Stamp
Downe, Kent	Royal College of Surgeons' Laboratory	J. C. Colbeck

[a] Closed by December 1941.
[b] Moved to Hill End Hospital, by December 1941.
[c] Moved to Middlesex Hospital, by December 1941.

Appendix Table 3 "Associated" laboratories, 1939–59[a]

Date	Laboratory	Location	Director	Subsequent history[b]
1939	Birmingham	Medical School	J. F. D. Shrewsbury	Ceased association 1947
	Leeds	Medical School	J. W. McLeod	CL (Seacroft), 1955
	Liverpool	City Bacteriology Laboratory	H. D. Wright D. T. Robinson (1943)	CL, 1955
	Manchester	University Public Health Laboratory	H. B. Maitland	CL, 1948
	Newcastle	Public Health Laboratory, Medical School	E. M. Dunlop S. H. Warren	CL, 1947
	Sheffield	University Department of Bacteriology	Wilson Smith	Municipal Laboratory 1946; CL, 1948
1940	Brighton	Hospital	L. R. Janes	CL, 1949
	Bristol	University Department of Preventive Medicine	K. E. Cooper	CL, 1959
	Cambridge	Private laboratory	W. Harvey	Ceased by 1946
	Carlisle	Hospital	J. S. Faulds	CL, 1955
	Dorchester	County Laboratory	T. V. Cooper	CL, 1951
	Eastbourne	Hospital	A. G. Shera	RL, 1950
	Hastings	Hospital	P. Lazarus Barlow	RL, 1950
	Peterborough	Hospital	D. H. Fulton	CL, 1946
	Plymouth	Hospital	E. Wordley	CL, 1953
	Poole	Municipal Laboratory	R. Archibald	CL, 1948
	Portsmouth	Hospital	J. A. D. Radcliffe	CL, 1949
	Reading	Hospital	J. Mills	CL, 1944
	Swansea	Hospital	A. F. Sladden	CL, 1956
	Worthing	Private laboratory	F. Standish	RL, 1950
1941	Birmingham	City Bacteriology Laboratory	H. Henry F. C. Lewis	CL, 1950
	Chichester	County Laboratory	F. Standish C. J. Harwood Little	Hospital, 1948; RL, 1950
	Salisbury	American Red Cross Hospital	J. E. Gordon	Ceased 1945
	Stafford	County Laboratory	J. L. Edwards	CL, 1947
	Wakefield	County Laboratory	P. L. Sutherland	CL, 1947
1942	Derby	County Laboratory	J. L. G. Iredale	CL, 1958
1943	Salisbury	Hospital	L. H. D. Thornton	CL, 1954

Appendix Table 3 (*contd*)

Date	Laboratory	Location	Director	Subsequent history[b]
1946	Maidstone[c]	County Laboratory	E. R. Jones	CL, 1955
	Newcastle/ Newburn	County Laboratory	A. I. Messer	CL, 1947
	Newcastle	City Bacteriology Laboratory	R. Norton	CL, 1947

[a] The dates quoted are the latest by which "associated" status was achieved; it was probably earlier in some cases

[b] *Abbreviations*: CL, constituent laboratory; RL, "recognized" laboratory (see p. 43)

[c] The Maidstone laboratory operated as an "associated" laboratory only for a number of special functions.

Appendix Table 4 "Recognized" laboratories

Date recognized	Laboratory	Date recognition ceased	Notes
Before 1950	Aylesbury, Stoke Mandeville	1972[a]	
	Chester, Royal Infirmary	(1960)[b]	
	Chichester, St Richard's Hospital	1951	Brighton and Portsmouth laboratories opened
	Ealing, King Edward Memorial Hospital	1961[c, d]	
	Eastbourne, Princess Alice Memorial Hospital	1954[e]	
	Gloucester, Royal Infirmary	(1964)[b]	
	Hastings, Royal East Sussex Hospital	1961[c, e]	
	Hellingly Hospital	1954[e]	
	Kettering and District Hospital	1961[c]	
	Sunderland, Royal Infirmary	(1950)[b]	
	Worthing, Shakespeare Road	1951[e]	Private laboratory
	York, County Hospital		
By 1951	Barrow, Group Pathology Laboratory	1960	Chester and Preston laboratories opened
	Blackburn, Royal Infirmary	1960	Chester and Preston laboratories opened
	Blackpool, Victoria Hospital	1960	Chester and Preston laboratories opened
	Bolton, Royal Infirmary	1972[a]	
	Burnley, Victoria Hospital	1960	Chester and Preston laboratories opened
	Lancaster, Royal Lancaster Infirmary	1965[c]	
	Oldham, Royal Infirmary	1960	Chester and Preston laboratories opened
	Preston, Royal Infirmary	(1958)[b]	
	Salford, Hope Hospital		Became a sub-laboratory to Manchester
	Stockport, Stepping Hill Hospital	1960	
	Wigan, Royal Infirmary	1972[a]	

[a] Not recorded in the PHLS Yearbook after this date.
[b] Became a constituent PHLS laboratory.
[c] Recognition ceased before the date given.
[d] Formerly a London Sector Emergency Public Health Laboratory.
[e] Formerly an "associated" laboratory.

Appendix Table 5 Developments in reference laboratories, 1949–79

Year	At Colindale	Elsewhere
1949	R. E. O. Williams appointed director of the Streptococcus and Staphylococcus Reference Laboratory National Collection of Type Cultures arrived (S. T. Cowan, Curator)	R. W. Riddell appointed director of the Mycological Reference Laboratory
1950		P. G. Shute appointed director of the Malaria Reference Laboratory
1952	Dysentery Reference Laboratory arrived (H. J. Bensted, director) New "tower block" opened	
1953	Air Hygiene Unit constituted	
1954	E. S. Anderson appointed director of the Enteric Reference Laboratory	Venereal Diseases Reference Laboratory transferred to the Eastern Hospital
1955		Venereal Diseases Reference Laboratory transferred to the London Hospital
1956	K. Patricia Carpenter appointed director of the Dysentery Reference Laboratory C. M. Patricia Bradstreet appointed director of the Standards Laboratory for Serological Reagents	
1959		Tuberculosis Reference Laboratory transferred to the PHLS (J. Marks, director) A. E. Wilkinson appointed director of the Venereal Diseases Reference Laboratory
1960	Cross-Infection Reference Laboratory formed from the Streptococcus and Staphylococcus Reference Laboratory and the Air Hygiene Unit (M. T. Parker, director) Disinfectant Reference Laboratory opened (J. C. Kelsey, director)	

Appendix Table 5 (*contd*)

Year	At Colindale	Elsewhere
1961	C. E. D. Taylor appointed director of the Routine Diagnostic Laboratory A. D. Macrae appointed director of the Virus Reference Laboratory J. C. McDonald appointed director of the Epidemiological Research Laboratory	Malaria Reference Laboratory transferred to the London School of Hygiene and Tropical Medicine I. G. Murray appointed director of the Mycological Reference Laboratory
1964	T. M. Pollock appointed director of the Epidemiological Research Laboratory S. P. Lapage appointed curator of the National Collection of Type Cultures	Leptospirosis Reference Laboratory opened at the London School of Hygiene and Tropical Medicine (L. Turner, director)
1967	Diagnostic Reference Laboratory closed	
1968	Edmonton sub-laboratory closed	
1970	B. Rowe appointed director of the Salmonella Reference Laboratory Marguerite S. Pereira appointed director of the Virus Reference Laboratory	
1971	Shigella Reference Laboratory merged with the Salmonella Reference Laboratory	Reference work on *Sh. sonnei* moved to Guildford laboratory
1972		D. W. R. Mackenzie appointed director of the Mycological Reference Laboratory
1973	Bacterial Metabolism Research Laboratory opened (R. E. O. Williams, director) Leptospirosis Reference Laboratory arrived	
1974		Microbiological Quality Control Laboratory opened (P. B. Crone, director)
1975	M. J. Hill appointed director of the Bacterial Metabolism Research Laboratory	
1976	Communicable Disease Surveillance Centre opened (N. S. Galbraith, director) R. J. Gilbert appointed director of the Food Hygiene Laboratory	Mycoplasma Reference Laboratory moved to Norwich laboratory

1977		Tuberculosis Reference Laboratory became the Mycobacterium Reference Unit (P. Jenkins, director) within the Cardiff laboratory
1978	Cross-Infection Laboratory became the Division of Hospital Infection (P. D. Meers, director) Salmonella and Shigella Reference Laboratory merged with the Enteric Reference Laboratory as the Division of Enteric Pathogens (B. Rowe, director) Leptospirosis Reference Laboratory became the Leptospira Reference Laboratory (Joyce Coglan, director) L. R. Hill appointed curator of the National Collection of Type Cultures	
1979	Standards Laboratory and Quality Control Laboratory merged as the Division of Microbiological Reagents and Quality Control (P. S. Gardner, director)	Nafra A. Johnson appointed acting director of the Venereal Diseases Reference Laboratory

Appendix Table 6 Revenue and capital expenditure, 1948–59 and 1961–80

Year	Expenditure (£)	
	Revenue	Capital
1948–49	537,880	39,631
1949–50	633,510	41,717
1950–51	779,648	87,634
1951–52	873,390	198,456
1952–53	857,157	155,620
1953–54	882,931	119,309
1954–55	934,923	99,508
1955–56	1,022,570	113,704
1956–57	1,092,114	97,525
1957–58	1,162,926	46,805
1958–59	1,164,851	36,404
1961–62	983,239	37,891
1962–63	1,581,237	65,662
1963–64	1,756,378	119,252
1964–65	1,838,923	176,901
1965–66	2,075,625	140,525
1966–67	2,273,911	155,521
1967–68	2,472,985	237,129
1968–69	2,740,440	426,726
1969–70	3,102,808	393,675
1970–71	3,676,608	228,028
1971–72	4,222,804	287,536
1972–73	4,785,257	517,230
1973–74	5,293,408	556,800
1974–75	7,166,291	459,446
1975–76	9,058,528	475,231
1976–77	10,413,020	612,829
1977–78	11,360,277	445,955
1978–79	12,905,281	1,023,641
1979–80	15,520,578	1,811,656

Notes: In 1950–1 the cost of reimbursements to "associated" and "recognized" laboratories was about £51,000. The proportion of the recurrent costs rechargeable to health authorities rose from £14,579 in 1961–2 to £1,030,031 in 1978–9.

Appendix Table 7 Members of the PHLS Boards, 1950–1980

MRC Board

A. Landsborough Thomson (Chairman), 1950–60[a]
S. P. Bedson, 1950–60
C. Metcalfe Brown, 1950–53
John A. Charles, 1950–60
A. N. Drury, 1950–53
P. Hartley, 1950–53
A. A. Miles, 1950–60[a]
W. H. Bradley (Observer), 1950–60
E. K. Macdonald, 1954–56
E. T. C. Spooner, 1954–60[a]
C. H. Stuart Harris, 1954–60[a]
G. W. H. Townsend, 1956–60

Statutory Board

A. Landsborough Thomson (Chairman), 1961–63
P. Alwyn Smith, 1961–65
A. H. Clough, 1961–67
A. W. Downie, 1961–67
E. Hughes, 1961–64
J. Stevenson Logan, 1961–67
J. R. McGregor, 1961–68
A. A. Miles, 1961–63
E. T. C. Spooner, 1961–72 (Chairman, 1964–72)
C. C. Stevens, 1961–
C. H. Stuart Harris, 1961–66
D. Thomson, 1961–65
G. I. Watson, 1963–75
A. C. Cunliffe, 1964–74
J. F. Warin, 1965–75
R. E. O. Williams, 1964–67
A. A. Driver, 1966–69
R. M. Shaw, 1966–74
N. P. L. Wildy, 1967–72
F. A. Adams, 1968–77
J. B. Meredith Davies, 1968–71
R. Knox, 1968–69
K. McCarthy, 1968–77
R. C. Bryant, 1969–75
A. J. Essex Cater, 1969–75
G. D. Duncan, 1970–75
R. A. Shooter, 1970–
C. E. Gordon Smith 1970– (Chairman, 1973–)
W. G. Harding, 1972–
D. G. Evans, 1973–74
H. M. Archibald, 1974–75
D. D. Reid, 1974–75
J. J. A. Reid, 1974
M. H. Richmond, 1974–
W. C. D. Lovett, 1975–
A. J. Rowland, 1975–
J. A. Scott, 1975–
S. Sherman, 1975–
E. L. Harris, 1977–
J. C. McDonald, 1977–80
W. O. Williams, 1977–
F. J. Aldridge, 1978–
W. F. J. Cuthbertson, 1978–80
T. H. Flewitt, 1978–
R. G. Hoare, 1978–

[a] Continued as a member of the Statutory Board.

Appendix Table 8 Committees, subcommittees and working parties set up by the Staff Committee, 1945–80[a]

Year	Topic of consideration
1945	Bacteriology of ice-cream
1946	Penicillin for treatment of diphtheria
	Chemotherapy of typhoid and paratyphoid fevers (penicillin and sulphathiazole)
1948	Bacteriological examination of shellfish
	Scarlet fever and streptococcal infections
	Salmonellas
	Diagnosis of tuberculosis
1949	Standardization of Widal test
	Revision of Memo 71 on bacteriological examination of water supplies
1950	Formaldehyde disinfection
1951	Brucella ring test
	Sonne dysentery
1953	Bacteriological contamination of bathing beaches
	Synthetic cream
	Spray-dried skim milk
1955	Bacteriological examination of waterworks employees
	Prevention of tuberculosis in laboratory workers
	Bacteriology of cream
	Viruses
1956	Food investigation
1957	Hospital infection
	Animal fertilizers and feedstuffs
	(Preliminary on farmers' lung)
1958	Atypical mycobacteria
1960	Salmonella in meat
1961	Testing and evaluation of disinfectants
	Watercress
1962	Non-bacterial enteritis
	Botulinum spores in cooked chicken
	Unusual acid-fast bacilli in lung lesions
	Autopsy survey of staphylococcal infection
	Hospital-acquired infection in medical wards
	Joint PHLS/MAFF on salmonellosis
1963	Antibiotic resistance of pathogens
	Protective cabinets
1964	Farmers' lung
	Bacteriological examination of water
	Refrigeration at −70 °C
	Brucellosis
1965	Virology
	Commercial culture media
	Immunofluorescent methods
	Rubella

Appendix Table 8 (*contd*)

Year	Topic of consideration
	Acute respiratory virus infections (with MRC) Joint PHLS/MAFF committee (on zoonoses)
1966	Whooping cough Bacteria in pharmaceutical products Routine sampling procedures
1967	Laboratory autoclaves Microbiological specifications for foods Viral reagents Bacteriological control of dialysis units
1968	Testing raw meat for salmonellae Hygiene of cream Streptococcal infections in residential schools
1969	Cytomegalovirus and immunofluorescence
1970	Quality control
1971	Hepatitis Installation and operation of centrifuges Influenza Brucella
1972	Bacteriological examination of water Influenza, with Royal College of General Practitioners
1974	Consideration of Cox recommendations on smallpox Virology in area laboratories (at request of PHLS Board)
1975	Laboratory safety Slaughterhouses (with MAFF) Laboratory autoclaves (PHLS Board established Advisory Committee of Microbiological Quality Control)
1976	Electron microscopy Zoonoses Panel (with MAFF) Salmonellas
1977	Serological reagents Standardization of methods for foods Communicable disease information (PHLS Board established Advisory Committee for Communicable Disease Surveillance Centre)
1978	Diagnosis of Legionnaires' disease Radial haemolysis for estimating rubella antibodies PHLS in relation to control of hospital infection
1979	Primary anoebic meningo-encephalitis
1980	Human infections with Group B streptococci Streptococcal infections in abattoir workers Campylobacter infections

[a] *Note*: The list is of topics rather than exact titles; it omits those committees set up for purely administrative matters.

Appendix Table 9 Technician/MLSO staff of the PHLS, 1953–79

Year	Number in technician or MLSO grades
1953	441
1958	507
1964	580
1975	802
1979	832

As indicated in the text there were, from the early years of the PHLS, a number of technicians employed by the hospital authorities working in the PHLS laboratories; the numbers concerned are not available until recent years; in 1979 there were 520 such MLSOs.

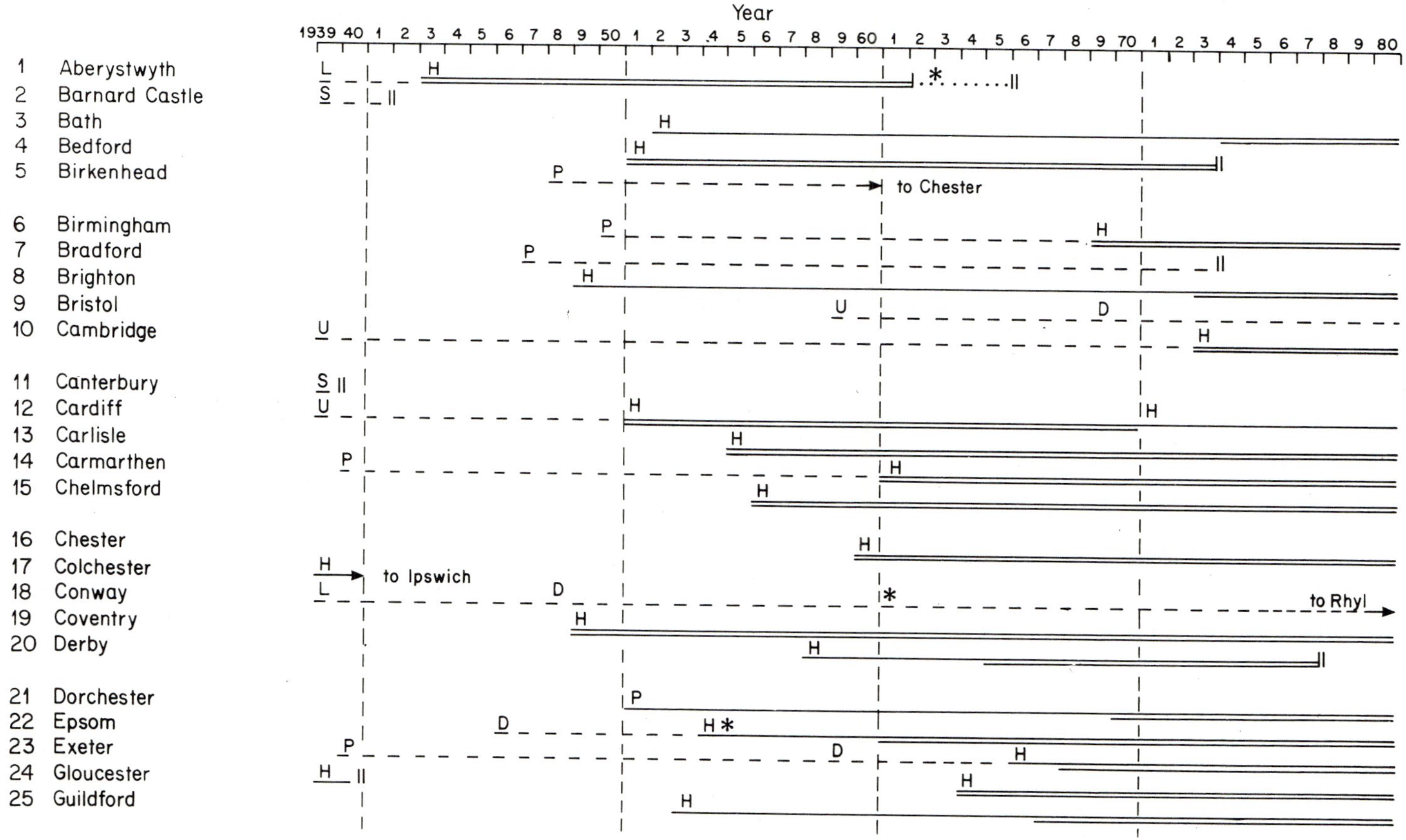

Appendix Figure 1 For caption see p. 202.

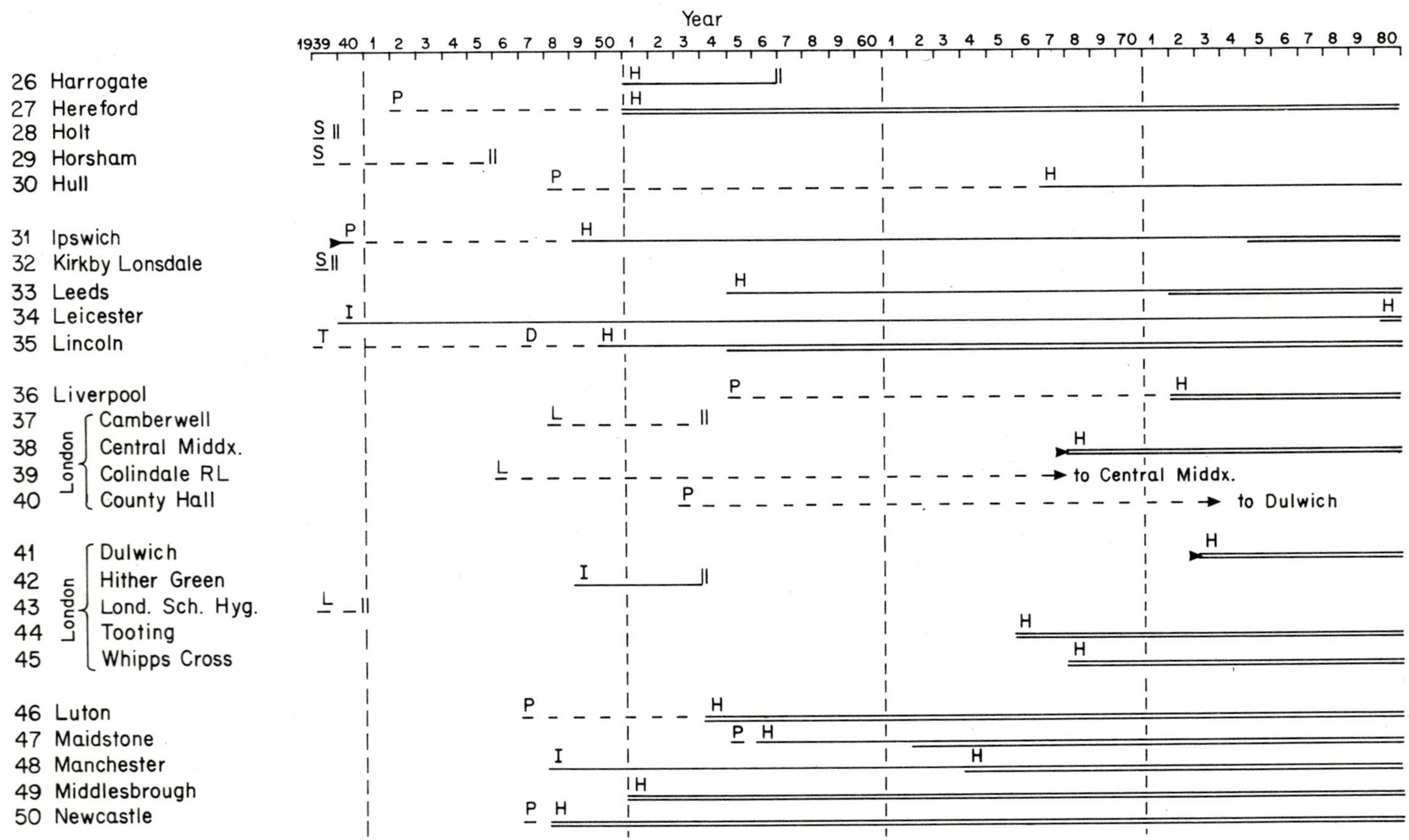

Year
1939 40 1 2 3 4 5 6 7 8 9 50 1 2 3 4 5 6 7 8 9 60 1 2 3 4 5 6 7 8 9 70 1 2 3 4 5 6 7 8 9 80
26 Harrogate
27 Hereford
28 Holt
29 Horsham
30 Hull
31 Ipswich
32 Kirkby Lonsdale
33 Leeds
34 Leicester
35 Lincoln
36 Liverpool
37 Camberwell
38 Central Middx.
39 Colindale RL
40 County Hall
London
41 Dulwich
42 Hither Green
43 Lond. Sch. Hyg.
44 Tooting
45 Whipps Cross
London
46 Luton
47 Maidstone
48 Manchester
49 Middlesbrough
50 Newcastle
to Central Middx.
to Dulwich

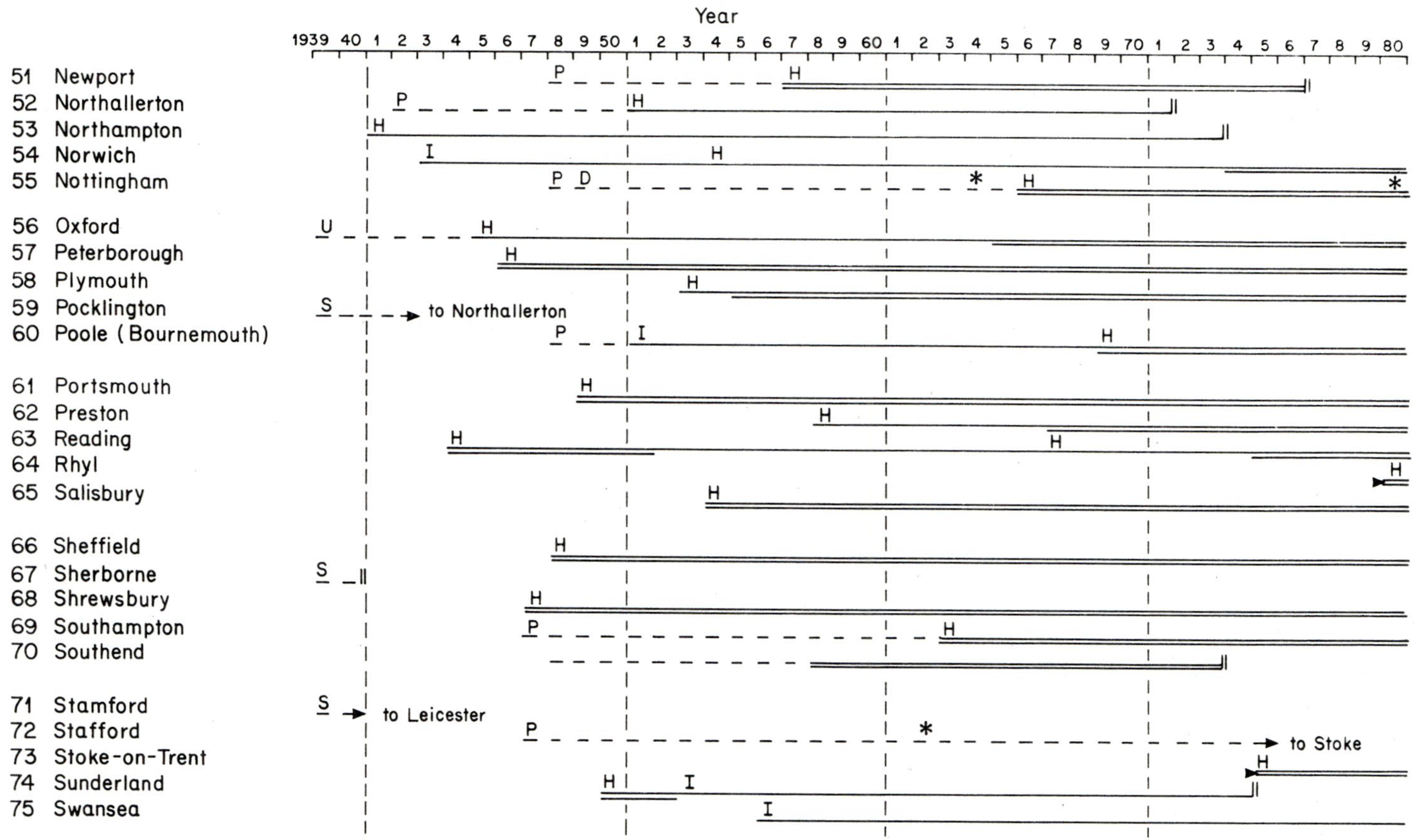

Appendix Figure 1 For caption see p. 202.

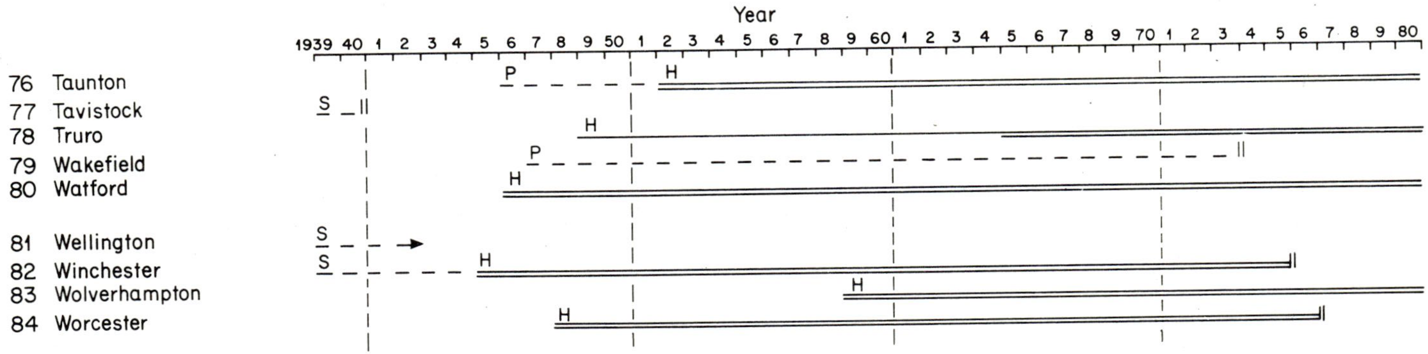

Appendix Figure 1 The constituent laboratories of the EPHLS and the PHLS, 1939–80. *Abbreviations*: L, various laboratories not in a hospital or a public health department; H, hospital; S, school; U, university; P, public health department; T, technical college; I, infectious diseases hospital or sanatorium; D, dedicated public health laboratory not in a hospital.

-----, laboratory not in a hospital; ——, laboratory in a hospital, but not doing general hospital work; ═══, laboratory in a hospital and doing general hospital work.

Asterisks indicate specific points at various laboratories as follows: Aberystwyth, technical presence retained; Conway, senior bacteriologist appointed for hospital work at Rhyl; Epsom, laboratory responsible for general hospital work but not situated in a general hospital; Nottingham, responsible for hospital at a distance from 1964, joint with university hospital from 1980; Stafford, off-site responsibility for hospital work.

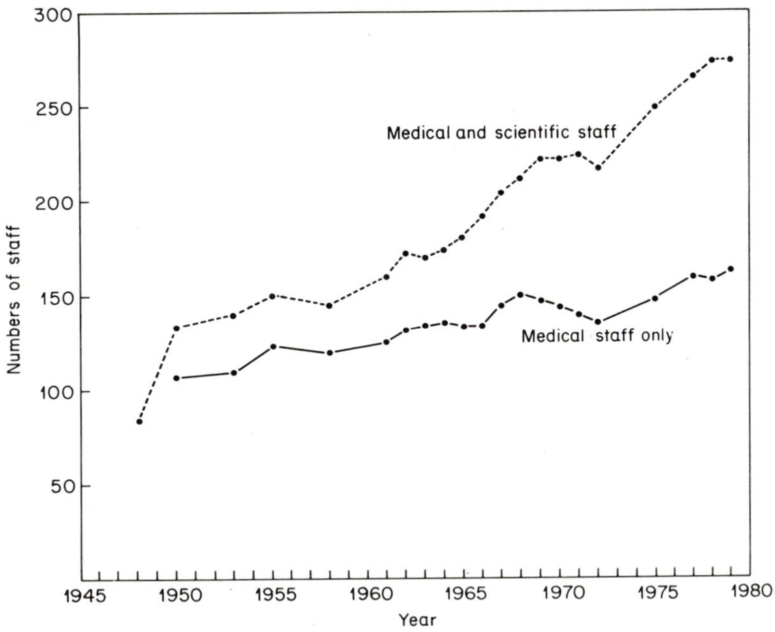

Appendix Figure 2 Medical and scientific staff of the PHLS, 1949–79. *Note*: the numbers refer to individuals, a few of whom worked part-time. "Scientific" staff numbers are those for graduate staff appointed as "scientific officers" and exclude those in medical laboratory scientific officer grades (see Appendix Table 9). In 1979 there were in addition 44 medical and nine scientific staff working in PHLS laboratories who were employed by regional or area health authorities.

References

Abbott, J.D., and Graves, J.F.R. (1972). Serotype and sulphonamide sensitivity of meningococci isolated from 1966 to 1971. *J. clin. Path.* **25**, 528.

Abbott, J.D., and Shannon, R. (1958). A method for typing *Shigella sonnei*, using colicine production as a marker. *J. clin. Path.* **11**, 71.

Allison, V.D., and Hobbs, B.C. (1947). An inquiry into the epidemiology of pemphigus neonatorum. *Br. med. J.* **2**, 1.

Anderson, E.S. (1959). Mutation in the type-determining phages of *Salmonella typhi*. *Nature, Lond.* **184**, 1822.

Anderson, E.S. (1965). Origin of transferable drug-resistance factors in the *Enterobacteriaceae*. *Br. med. J.* **2**, 1289.

Anderson, E.S. (1975). The problem and implications of chloramphenicol resistance in the typhoid bacillus. *J. Hyg., Camb.* **74**, 289.

Anderson, E.S., and Hobbs B.C. (1973). Studies of the strain of *Salmonella typhi* responsible for the Aberdeen typhoid outbreak. *Israel J. med. Sci.* **9**, 162.

Anderson, E.S., Ward, L.R., De Saxe, M.J., Old, D.C., Barker, R., and Duguid, J.P. (1978). Correlation of phage type, biotype and source in strains of *Salmonella typhimurium*. *J. Hyg., Camb.* **81**, 203.

Andrews, B.E., Beare, A.S., McDonald, J.C., Zuckerman, A.J., and Tyrell, D.A.J. (1966). Further trials of live influenza vaccine. *Br. med. J.* **1**, 637.

Anon. (1944). William Whiteman Carlton Topley: obituary. *Lancet i*, 198.

Anon. ("A provincial pathologist") (1958). [Letter to the Editor.] *Lancet i*, 799.

Apley, J., Clarke, S.K.R., Roome, A.P.C.H., Sandry, S.A., Saygi, G., Silk, B., and Warhurst, D.C. (1970). Primary amoebic meningoencephalitis in Britain. *Br. med. J.* **1**, 596.

Appleton, H., Buckley, M., Thom, B.T., Cotton, J.L., and Henderson, S. (1977). Virus-like particles in winter vomiting disease. *Lancet i*, 409.

Appleton, H., and Pereira, M.S. (1977). A possible virus aetiology in outbreaks of food poisoning from cockles. *Lancet i*, 780.

Asheshov, E.H. (1969). The genetics of penicillinase production in *Staphylococcus aureus* strain PS80. *J. gen. Microbiol.* **59**, 289.

Barrow, G.I., and Miller, D.C. (1972). *Vibrio parahaemolyticus*: a potential pathogen from marine sources in Britain. *Lancet i*, 485.

Bartlett, C.L.R. (1979). Sporadic cases of Legionnaires' disease in Great Britain. *Ann. intern. Med.* **90**, 592.

Bashford, T.E., Gillespy, T.G., and Tomlinson, A.J.H. (1960). "Staphylococcal Food Poisoning Associated with Processed Peas". Chipping Campden: The Fruit and Vegetable Canning and Quick Freezing Research Association.

Bassett, D.C.J. (1971). Causes and prevention of sepsis due to Gram-negative bacteria: common source outbreaks. *Proc. R. Soc. Med.* **64**, 980.

Bettelheim, K.A., Dulake, C., and Taylor, J. (1971). Post-operative urinary infections caused by *Escherichia coli*. *J. clin. Path.* **24**, 442.

Bevan, G., Evans, R., Pugh, I., Sudds, M.V.N., Parker, M.T., and Sladden, A.F.S. (1948). Penicillin and sulphathiazole in typhoid fever. *Lancet i*, 545.

Blowers, R., and Crew, B. (1960). Ventilation of operating theatres. *J. Hyg., Camb.* **58**, 427.

Blowers, R., and McCluskey, M. (1965). Design of operating room dress for surgeons. *Lancet ii*, 681.

Blowers, R., Mason, G.A., Wallace, K.R., and Walton, M. (1955). Control of wound infection in a thoracic surgery unit. *Lancet ii*, 786.

Boissard, G.P.B., Stokes, L.J., Macrae, A.D., and MacCallum, F.O. (1957). Isolation of viruses related to Echo virus type 9 from outbreaks of aseptic meningitis. *Lancet i*, 500.

Bourdillon, R.B., Lidwell, O.M., and Lovelock, J.E. (1948). Studies in air hygiene. *Spec. Rep. Ser, med. Res. Coun., Lond.* No. 262.

Bradley, W.H. (1943). Epidemiological study of *Bact. typhosum* type D4. *Br. med. J.* **1**, 438.

Bradstreet, C.M.P., Pereira, M.S., and Andrews, B.E. (1964). The development of a national virological diagnosis service. *Prog. med. Virol.* **6**, 149.

Bray, J. (1945). Isolation of antigenically homogeneous strains of *Bact. coli neapolitanum* from summer diarrhoea of infants. *J. Path. Bact.* **57**, 239.

British Medical Bulletin (1951). Public Health Laboratory Service. *Br. med. Bull.* **7**, 147.

Bullen, C.L., and Willis, A.T. (1971). Resistance of the breast-fed infant to gastroenteritis. *Br. med. J.* **3**, 338.

Callow, B.R. (1959). A new phage-typing scheme for *Salmonella typhi-murium*. *J. Hyg., Camb.* **57**, 346.

Caul, E.O., and Clarke, S.K.R. (1975). Coronavirus propagated from patient with non-bacterial gastroenteritis. *Lancet ii*, 953.

Clarke, S.K.R., Cook, G.T., Egglestone, S.I., Hall, T.S., Miller, D.L., Reed, S.E., Rubenstein, D., Smith, A.J., and Tyrell, D.A.J. (1972). A virus from epidemic vomiting disease. *Br. med. J.* **3**, 86.

Clifford, R.E., Smith, J.W.G., Tillett, H.E., and Wherry, P.J. (1977). Excess mortality associated with influenza in England and Wales. *Int. J. Epidem.* **6**, 115.

Cockburn, W.C. (1955). Large-scale field trials of active immunizing agents, with special reference to vaccination against pertussis. *Bull. Wld Hlth Org.* **13**, 395.

Cockburn, W.C., and Holt, H.D. (1948). A comparison of the results obtained with pernasal and postnasal swabs in the diagnosis of pertussis. *Mon. Bull. Min. Hlth Lab. Serv.* **7**, 156.

Cockburn, W.C., Harrington, J.A., Zeitlin, R.A., Morris, D., and Camps, F.E. (1951). Homologous serum hepatitis and measles prophylaxis. *Br. med. J.* **2**, 6.

Cockburn, W.C., Jameson, J.E., and Fenton, J. (1951). An explosive outbreak of paratyphoid B fever due to Vi-phage type "Taunton". *Mon. Bull. Min. Hlth Lab. Serv.* **10**, 43, 49.

Collins, C.H. (1953). Differences between tubercle bacilli and other acid fast bacilli from human sources. *Acta tuberc. scand.* **28**, 340.

Couper, W.R.M., Newell, K.W., and Payne, D.J.H. (1956). An outbreak of typhoid fever associated with canned ox-tongue. *Lancet i*, 1057.

Cradock-Watson, J.E., Ridehalgh, M.K.S., and Chantler, S. (1976). Specific immunoglobulins in infants with the congenital rubella syndrome. *J. Hyg., Camb.* **76**, 109.

Craske, J., Kirk, P., Cohen, B.J., and Vandervelde, E.M. (1978). Commercial factor VIII associated with hepatitis, 1974–75 in the United Kingdom: a retrospective survey. *J. Hyg., Camb.* **80**, 327.

Cruickshank, J.C. (1947). Typhoid fever in Devon. The value of phage-typing in a rural area. *Mon. Bull. Min. Hlth Lab. Serv.* **6**, 88.

Dillon, H.C., Moody, M.D., Maxted, W.R., and Parker, M.T. (1967). The epidemiology of impetigo and acute glomerulonephritis: results of serological typing of group A streptococci. *Am. J. Epidem.* **86**, 710.

Dyke, S.C., (1961). In Foster (1961), q.v.

Edgar, W.M. (1965). The PHLS [Letter to the Editor]. *Lancet i*, 599.

Edwards, J.M.B., and Woodruff, M. (1979). EB virus-specific IgA in serum of patients with infectious mononucleosis and of healthy people of different ages. *J. clin. Path.* **32**, 1036.

Evans, A.D. (1956). Q fever in South Wales. *Mon. Bull. Min. Hlth Lab. Serv.* **15**, 215.

Felix, A. (1941). A new type of typhoid and paratyphoid vaccine. *Br. med. J.* **1**, 391.
Felix, A. (1943). Experiences with typing typhoid bacilli by means of Vi bacteriophage. *Br. med. J.* **1**, 435.
Ferguson, I.R., and Tearle, P.V. (1977). Gas liquid chromatography in the rapid diagnosis of meningitis. *J. clin. Path.* **30**, 1163.
Fisher-Hoch, S.P., Hudson, M.J., and Thompson, M.H. (1979). Identification of a clinical isolate as *Legionella pheumophila* by gas chromatography and mass spectometry of cellular fatty acids. *Lancet ii*, 323.
Flewett, T.H., Bryden, A.S., and Davies, H. (1973). Virus particles in gastroenteritis [Letter to the Editor]. *Lancet ii*, 1497.
Foster, W.D. (1961). "A Short History of Clinical Pathology". London: Churchill.
Fraser, C.A.M., Ball, L.C., Morris, C.A., and Noah, N.D. (1977). Serological characterization of group-A streptococci associated with skin sepsis in meat handlers. *J. Hyg., Camb.* **78**, 283.
Fulton, F., Taylor, J., Wells, A.Q., and Wilson, G.S. (1941). Combined active and passive immunization against diphtheria. II. Control of epidemics in the field. *Br. med. J.* **2**, 759.
Galbraith, N.S. (1966). A survey of poliovirus excretion in normal children, England and Wales 1961–1962. *Proc. X Symp. Europ. Assoc. Polio., Warsaw 1964.* Paris: Masson, p. 119.
Galpine, J.F., and Macrae, A.D. (1953). An outbreak of benign meningo-encephalitis: isolation of Coxsackie virus. *Lancet i*, 372.
Geffen, T.J., and Spicer, C.C. (1960). Poliomyelitis in the vaccinated: England and Wales 1958. *Lancet ii*, 87.
Gilbert, R.J., and Parry, J.M. (1977). Serotypes of *Bacillus cereus* from outbreaks of food poisoning and from routine foods. *J. Hyg., Camb.* **78**, 69.
Gilbert, R.S., Wieneke, A.A., Lausaer J., and Šimkovičová, M. (1972). Serological detection of enterotoxin in foods implicated in staphylococcal food poisoning. *J. Hyg., Camb.* **70**, 755.
Goffe, A.P., Beveridge, J.J., and MacCallum, F.O. (1960). Poliomyelitis virus in sewage. *Mon. Bull. Min. Hlth Lab. Serv.* **19**, 9.
Goodburn, G.M., and Marmion, B.P. (1962). A study of the properties of Eaton's primary atypical pneumonia organism. *J. gen. Microbiol.* **29**, 271.
Grist, N.R. (1975). Hepatitis in clinical laboratories: a three-year survey. *J. clin. Path.* **28**, 255.
Hambling, M.H. (1980). Changes in the distribution of rubella antibodies in women of child-bearing age during the first eight years of a rubella vaccination programme. *J. Infect.* **2**, 341.
Harvey, R.W.S., Price, T.H., Foster, D.W., and Griffiths, W.C. (1969). Salmonellas in sewage: a study in latent human infection. *J. Hyg., Camb.* **67**, 517.
Higgins, P.G. (1974). Viruses associated with acute respiratory infections, 1961–71. *J. Hyg., Camb.* **72**, 425.
Hill, L.R. (1974). Theoretical aspects of numerical identification. *Int. J. syst. Bact.* **24**, 494.
Hobbs, B.C. (1965). *Clostridium welchii* as a food poisoning organism. *J. appl. Bact.* **28**, 74.
Hobbs, B.C., Rowe, B., Kendall, M., Turnbull, P.C.B., and Ghosh, A.C. (1976). *Escherichia coli* 027 in adult diarrhoea. *J. Hyg., Camb.* **77**, 393.
Hobbs, B.C., Smith, M.E., Oakley, C.L., Warrack, G.H., and Cruickshank, J.C. (1953). *Clostridium welchii* food poisoning. *J. Hyg., Camb.* **51**, 75.
Holmes, M.C., and Williams, R.E.O. (1954). The distribution of carriers of *Streptococcus pyogenes* among 2,413 healthy children. *J. Hyg., Camb.* **52**, 165.
Holmes, M.C., and Williams, R.E.O. (1958). Streptococcal infections among children in a residential home. *J. Hyg., Camb.* **56**, 43, 62, 197, 211.
Hooper, W.L., Barrow, G.I., and McNab, D.J.N. (1974). *Vibrio parahaemolyticus* food poisoning in Britain. *Lancet i*, 1100.
Hoskins, T.W., Davies, J.R., Smith, A.J., Miller, C.L., and Allchin, A. (1979). Assessment of inactivated influenza-A vaccine after three outbreaks of influenza A at Christ's Hospital. *Lancet i*, 33.
Howie, J.W. (1965*a*). The Public Health Laboratory Service. *Lancet i*, 501.

Howie, J.W. (1965*b*). The PHLS [Letter to the Editor]. *Lancet i*, 651.
Howie, J.W. (1970). Democratic direction. *Br. med. J.* **4**, 793.
Howie, J.W., and Timbury, Morag, C. (1956). Laboratory tests of operating theatre sterilisers. *Lancet ii*, 669.
Hoyle, L. (1941). A tellurite blood–agar medium for the rapid diagnosis of diphtheria. *Lancet i*, 175.
Hoyle, L. (1952). The multiplication of complement-fixing antigen and red-cell agglutinin in the chorio-allantoic membrane of fertile eggs inoculated with influenza virus. *J. Path. Bact.* **64**, 419.
Hoyle, L. (1954). The release of influenza virus from the infected cell. *J. Hyg., Camb.* **52**, 180.
Hoyle, L. (1968). "The Influenza Viruses" (Virology Monograph No. 4). Wien: Springer-Verlag.
Hoyle, L., and Frisch-Niggemeyer, W. (1955). The disintegration of influenza virus particles on entry into the host cell: studies with virus labelled with radiophosphorus. *J. Hyg., Camb.* **53**, 474.
Jellard, J. (1957). Umbilical cord as a reservoir of infection in a maternity hospital. *Br. med. J.* **1**, 925.
Jenkins, P.A. (1981*a*). Lipid analysis for the identification of mycobacteria: an appraisal. *Rev. infect. Dis.* **3**, 1021.
Jenkins, P.A. (1981*b*). The epidemiology of opportunist mycobacterial infections in Wales, 1952–1978. *Rev. infect. Dis.* **3**, 862.
Jevons, M.P., and Parker, M.T. (1964). The evolution of new hospital strains of *Staphylococcus aureus*. *J. clin. Path.* **17**, 243.
Johnston, H.H., Mitchell, C.J., and Curtis, G.D.W. (1976). An automated test for the detection of significant bacteriuria. *Lancet ii*, 400.
Jones, D.M., and Eldridge, J. (1981). Meningococcal disease in England and Wales 1978–79: a change in the serotype pattern. *J. Infect.* **3**, 134.
Joynson, D.H.M., Howells, C.H.L., Liddington, R., and Williams, A. (1975). Contamination of fluids from a hospital pharmacy. *J. Hyg., Camb.* **75**, 87.
Kass, E.H. (1956). Asymptomatic infection of the urinary tract. *Trans. Ass. Am. Physicians* **69**, 56.
Kendall, E.J.C., Riddle, R.W., Tuck, H.A., Rodan, K.S., Andrews, B.E., and McDonald, J.C. (1957). Pharyngo-conjunctival fever: school outbreaks in England during the summer of 1955 associated with adenovirus types 3, 7 and 14. *Br. med. J.* **2**, 131.
Knox, R. (1944). Comparison of Loeffler's inspissated serum and tellurite blood medium in the laboratory diagnosis of diphtheria. *Mon. Bull. Min. Hlth Lab. Serv.* **3**, 121.
Lapage, S.P., Bascomb, S., Willcox, W.R., and Curtis, M.A. (1973). Identification of bacteria by computer: general aspects and perspectives. *J. gen. Microbiol.* **77**, 273.
Lee, J.A. (1974). Recent trends in human salmonellosis in England and Wales: the epidemiology of prevalent serotypes other than *Salmonella typhimurium*. *J. Hyg., Camb.* **72**, 185.
Lidwell, O.M. (1959), Impaction sampler for size grading air-borne bacteria-carrying particles. *J. scient. Instrum.* **36**, 3.
Lidwell, O.M. (1961). Sepsis in surgical wounds: multiple regression analysis applied to records of post-operative hospital sepsis. *J. Hyg., Camb.* **59**, 259.
Lidwell, O.M., and Towers, A.G. (1972). Unidirectional (laminar) flow ventilation for patient isolation. *Lancet i*, 347.
Lidwell, O.M., Brock, B., Shooter, R.A., Cooke, E.M., and Thomas, G.E. (1975). Airborne infection in a fully air-conditioned hospital. IV. Airborne dispersal of *Staphylococcus aureus* and its nasal acquisition by patients. *J. Hyg., Camb.* **75**, 445.
Lidwell, O.M., Davies, J., Payne, R.W., Newman, P., and Williams, R.E.O. (1971). Nasal acquisition of *Staphylococcus aureus* in partly divided wards. *J. Hyg., Camb.* **69**, 113.
Lidwell, O.M., Polakoff, S., Davies, J., Hewitt, J.M., Shooter, R.A., Walker, K.A., Gaya, H., and Taylor, G.W. (1970). Nasal acquisition of *Staphylococcus aureus* in a subdivided and mechanically ventilated ward: endemic prevalence of a single staphyloccal strain. *J. Hyg., Camb.* **68**, 417.

Limentani, A.E., Elliott, L.M., Noah, N.D., and Lamborn, J.K. (1979). An outbreak of hepatitis B from tattooing. *Lancet ii*, 86.

Luton and Dunstable Hospital (1974). Metronidazole in the prevention and treatment of bacteroides infections in gynaecological patients. *Lancet ii*, 1540.

Luton and Dunstable Hospital (1975). An evaluation of metronidazole in the prophylaxis and treatment of anaerobic infections in surgical patients. *J. antimicrob. Chemother,* **1**, 393.

MRC (1947). The bacteriology of spray-dried egg with particular reference to food-poisoning. *Spec. Rep. Ser. med. Res. Coun., Lond.* No. 260.

MRC (1951). The prevention of whooping-cough by vaccination. *Br. med. J.* **2**, 1207.

MRC (1956). Poliomyelitis and prophylactic inoculation against diphtheria, whooping-cough, and smallpox. *Lancet ii*, 1223.

MRC (1962). Design and ventilation of operating-room suites for control of infection and for comfort. *Lancet ii*, 945.

MRC and PHLS (1980). The incidence of hepatitis B infection after accidental exposure and anti-HBs immunoglobulin prophylaxis [a combined MRC and PHLS report]. *Lancet i*, 6.

MacCallum, F.O. (1952). Laboratory diagnosis of smallpox. *J.R. sanit. Inst.* **72**, 112.

MacCallum, F.O., and McDonald, J.R. (1957). Survival of variola virus in raw cotton. *Bull. Wld Hlth Org.* **16**, 247.

MacCallum, F.O., McFarlan, A.M., Miles, J.A.R., and Wilson, C. (1951). Infective hepatitis studies in East Anglia during the period 1943–47. *Spec. Rep. Ser. med. Res. Coun., Lond.* No. 273.

MacCallum, F.O., Marmion, B.P., and Stoker, M.G.P. (1949). Q fever in Great Britain: isolation of *Rickettsia burneti* from an indigenous case. *Lancet ii*, 1026.

McConnell, M.M., Smith, H.R., Leonardopoulos, J., and Anderson, E.S. (1979). The value of plasmid studies in the epidemiology of infections due to drug-resistant *Salmonella wien. J. infect. Dis.* **139**, 178.

McCoy, J.R. (1975). Trends in salmonella food poisoning in England and Wales 1941–72. *J. Hyg., Camb.* **74**, 271.

McFarlan, A.M., Topley, E., and Fisher, M. (1945). Trial of whooping-cough vaccine in city and residential nursery groups. *Br. med. J.* **2**, 205.

Macrae, A.D., and Lewis, M.J. (1977). Legionnaires' disease in Nottingham [Letter to the Editor]. *Lancet ii*, 1225.

Mair, N.S., Mair, H.J., Stirk, E.M., and Corson, J.G. (1960). Three cases of acute mesenteric lymphadenitis due to *Pasteurella pseudotuberculosis. J. clin. Path.* **13**, 432.

Marks, J. (1961). The design of sensitivity tests on tubercle bacilli. *Tubercle, Lond.* **42**, 314.

Marks, J. (1965). Bacteriological aspects of the National Register of drug-resistant tuberculosis in its first two years. *Mon. Bull. Min. Hlth Lab. Serv.* **24**, 2.

Marks, J. (1969). "Opportunist" mycobacteria in England and Wales. *Tubercle, Lond.* **50** (Suppl.), 78.

Marks, J. (1972). Classification of the mycobacteria in relation to clinical significance. *Tubercle, Lond.* **53**, 259.

Marks, J. (1976). A system for the examination of tubercle bacilli and other mycobacteria. *Tubercle, Lond.* **57**, 207.

Marmion, B.P., and Stoker, M.G.P. (1958). The epidemiology of Q fever in Great Britain. *Br. med. J.* **2**, 809.

Marples, R.R., Hone, R., Notley, C.M., Richardson, J.P., and Crees-Morris, J.A. (1978). Investigation of coagulase-negative staphylococci from infections in a cardiac surgery unit. *Proc. Soc. gen. Microbiol.* **5**, 77.

Maxted, W.R., and Valkenburg, H.A. (1969). Variation in the M-antigen of group-A streptococci. *J. med. Microbiol.* **2**, 199.

Maxted, W.R., Widdowson, J.P., Fraser, C.A.M., Ball, L.C., and Bassett, D.C.J. (1972). The use of the serum opacity reaction in the typing of group-A streptococci. *J. med. Microbiol.* **6,** 83.

Miller, D.L. (1973). Collaborative studies of acute respiratory disease in patients seen in general practice, and in children admitted to hospital: aims, field methods and morbidity rates. *Postgrad. med. J.* **49**, 749.

Miller, D.L., and Galbraith, N.S. (1965). Surveillance of the safety of oral poliomyelitis vaccine in England and Wales 1962–4. *Br. med. J.* **2**, 504.

Miller, D.L., and Lee, J.A. (1969). Influenza in Britain 1967–68. *J. Hyg., Camb.* **67**, 559.

Moore, B. (1948). The detection of paratyphoid carriers in towns by means of sewage examination. *Mon. Bull. Min. Hlth Lab. Serv.* **7**, 241.

Moore, B. (1963). Methods of ascertainment. In "Infection in Hospitals: Epidemiology and Control" (CIOMS Symposium), R.E.O. Williams and R.A. Shooter (eds). Oxford: Blackwell, p. 7.

Mortimer, P.P., Vandervelde, E.M., and Parry, J.V. (1979). Serological evidence for recent infection with hepatitis A virus (HAV) following an institutional outbreak of hepatitis. *J. Infect.* **1**, 269.

Mortimer, P.R., and McCann, G. (1974). Food poisoning episodes associated with *Bacillus cerus* in fried rice. *Lancet i*, 1043.

Murray, L.H., and Bradley, W.H. (1948). Smallpox in 1947. *Mon. Bull. Min. Hlth Lab. Serv.* **7,** 96.

Nagington, J. (1964). Electron microscopy in differential diagnosis of poxvirus infections. *Br. med. J.* **2**, 1499.

National Collection of Type Cultures (1971). "The First Fifty Years: 1920–1970". London: PHLS.

Noah, N.D., and Urquart, A.M. (1980*a*). Virus meningitis and encephalitis in 1979. *J. Infect*, **2**, 379.

Noah, N.D., and Urquart, A.M. (1980*b*). Epidemiology of *Mycoplasma pneumoniae* infection in the British Isles, 1974–9. *J. Infect.* **2**, 191.

Nuffield Provincial Hospitals Trust (1958). "Present Sterilizing Practices in Six Hospitals". London: Nuffield Provincial Hospitals Trust.

PHLS (1948). Penicillin in diphtheria. *Lancet ii*, 517.

PHLS (1949*a*). Non-pulmonary tuberculosis in England and Wales: an account of a group investigation undertaken during the years 1943 to 1945. *J. Hyg., Camb.* **47**, 337.

PHLS (1949*b*). The bacteriological examination and grading of ice-cream. *Mon. Bull. Min. Hlth Lab. Serv.* **8**, 155.

PHLS (1950). Gamma globulin in the prevention and attenuation of measles: controlled trials in day and residential nurseries. *Lancet ii*, 732.

PHLS (1954). A field investigation of PTAP (purified toxoid, aluminium-phosphate-precipitated). *Mon. Bull. Min. Hlth Lab. Serv.* **13**, 127.

PHLS (1956*a*). A comparison of the Aschaffenburg–Mullen and Kay–Graham tests for phosphatase in milk. *Mon. Bull. Min. Hlth Lab. Serv.* **15**, 65.

PHLS (1956*b*). The value of the milk ring test (M.R.T.) and related tests in the detection of brucella organisms in milk supplies. *Mon. Bull. Min. Hlth Lab. Serv.* **15**, 85.

PHLS (1958*a*). The contamination of egg products with salmonellae, with particular reference to *Salm. paratyphi* B. *Mon. Bull. Min. Hlth Lab. Serv.* **17**, 36.

PHLS (1958*b*). Disinfection of fabrics with gaseous formalydehyde. *J. Hyg., Camb.* **56**, 488.

PHLS (1958*c*). Precautions against tuberculosis infection in the diagnostic laboratory. *Mon. Bull. Min. Hlth Lab. Serv.* **17**, 10.

PHLS (1958*d*). Deaths from Asian influenza, 1957. *Br. med. J.* **1**, 915.

PHLS (1958*e*). The incidence of poliomyelitis virus in normal children under 5 years. *Mon. Bull. Min. Hlth Lab. Serv.* **17**, 231.

PHLS (1958*f*). Report on examination of home contacts of poliomyelitis. *Mon. Bull. Min. Hlth Lab. Serv.* **17**, 58.

PHLS (1958*g*). The bacteriological examination and grading of fresh cream. *Mon. Bull. Min. Hlth Lab. Serv.* **17**, 77.

PHLS (1959*a*). Sewage contamination of bathing waters in England and Wales. *J. Hyg., Camb.* **57**, 435.

PHLS (1959*b*). Salmonella organisms in animal feeding stuffs and fertilizers. *Mon. Bull. Min. Hlth Lab. Serv.* **18**, 26.

PHLS (1960). Incidence of surgical wound infection in England and Wales. *Lancet ii*, 659.

PHLS (1961*a*). Trial of living attenuated poliovirus vaccine. *Br. med. J.* **2**, 1037.

PHLS(1961*b*). *Brucella abortus* in milk in England and Wales in 1959. *Mon. Bull. Min. Hlth Lab. Serv.* **20**, 33.

PHLS (1961*c*). Drug resistance in untreated pulmonary tuberculosis in England and Wales during 1960. *Tubercle, Lond.* **42**, 308.

PHLS (1965*a*). Infections acquired in medical wards. *J. Hyg., Camb.* **63**, 457.

PHLS (1965*b*). Whooping cough in Manchester, 1963–64. *Mon. Bull. Min. Hlth Lab. Serv.* **24**, 104.

PHLS (1966). Necropsy survey of staphylococcal infection on patients dying in hospitals. *Br. med. J.* **1**, 313.

PHLS (1967). Coxsackie B5 virus infections during 1965. *Br. med. J.* **4**, 575.

PHLS (1968). Infection risks of haemodialysis: some preventive aspects. *Br. med. J.* **3**, 454.

PHLS (1969). Efficacy of vaccines used in the United Kingdom before 1968. *Br. med. J.* **4**, 329.

PHLS (1970). Studies of the effect of immunoglobulin on rubella in pregnancy. *Br. med. J.* **2**, 497.

PHLS (1971). Infectious mononucleosis and its relationship to EB virus antibody [A joint investigation by university health physicians and PHLS laboratories]. *Br. med. J.* **4**, 643.

PHLS (1975). A programme for collaborative influenza surveillance. *J. Hyg., Camb.* **75**, 1.

PHLS (1976*a*). Survey on colony counts and predominant organisms in samples of boiled and fried rice from Chinese and Indian restaurants and "take-away" shops. *Environm. Hlth* **84**, 141.

PHLS (1976*b*). Hepatitis B in retreat from dialysis units in the United Kingdom in 1973. *Br. med. J.* **1**, 1579.

PHLS (1977). Influenza surveillance 1972–75. *J. Hyg., Camb.* **78**, 223.

PHLS (1980*a*). Salmonella infections in hospitals. *J. Hosp. Infect.* **1**, 307.

PHLS (1980*b*). Acute hepatitis B associated with gynaecological surgery. *Lancet ii*, 337.

PHLS, Skovgaarde, N., and Nielsen, B.B. (1972). Salmonellas in pigs and animal feeding stuffs in England and Wales and in Denmark. *J. Hyg., Camb.* **70**, 127.

Parker, M.T. (1969). Postoperative clostridial infections in Britain. *Br. med. J.* **3**, 671.

Parker, M.T. (1979). Infections with group-B streptococci. *J. antimicrob. Chemother.* **5** (Suppl. A), 27.

Parker, M.T., and Ball, L.C. (1976). Streptococci and aerococci associated with systemic infection in man. *J. med. Microbiol.* **9**, 275.

Parker, M.T., Tomlinson, A.J.H., and Williams, R.E.O. (1955). Impetigo contagiosa: the association of certain types of *Staphylococcus aureus* and of *Streptococcus pyogenes* with superficial skin infections. *J. Hyg., Camb.* **53**, 458.

Parker, M.T., Asheshov, E.H., Hewitt, J.H., Nakhla, L.S., and Brock, B.M. (1974). Endemic staphylococcal infections in hospitals. *Ann. N.Y. Acad. Sci.* **236**, 466.

Payne, D.J.H., and Scudamore, J.M. (1977). Outbreaks of salmonella food-poisoning over a period of eight years from a common source. *Lancet ii*, 1249.

Pereira, M.S., and Chakraverty, P. (1977). The laboratory surveillance of influenza epidemics in the United Kingdom, 1968–1976. *J. Hyg., Camb.* **79**, 77.

Pereira, M.S., Chakraverty, P., Schild, G.C., Coleman, M.T., and Dowdle, W.R. (1972). Prevalence of antibody to current influenza viruses and effect of vaccination on antibody response. *Br. med. J.* **4**, 701.

Perks, E.M., and Mayon-White, R.T. (1983). The incidence of scarlet fever. *J. Hyg., Camb.* **91**, 203.

Phillips, I. (1976). Beta-lactamase-producing, penicillin-resistant gonococcus. *Lancet ii*, 656.

Pitt, T.L., and Bradley, D.E. (1975). The antibody response to the flagella of *Pseudomonas aeruginosa*. *J. med. Microbiol*, **8**, 97.

Pitt, T.L., Erdman, Y.J., and Bucher, C. (1980). The epidemiological type identification of *Serratia marcescens* from outbreaks of infection in hospitals. *J. Hyg., Camb.* **84**, 269.

Polakoff, S. (1974). Decrease in the incidence of hepatitis in dialysis units associated with the prevention programme. *Br. med. J.* **4**, 751.

Polakoff, S., Cossart, Y.E., and Tillett, H.E. (1972). Hepatitis in dialysis units in the United Kingdom. *Br. med. J.* **3**, 94.

Reid, D.D. (1957). Incidence of tuberculosis among workers in medical laboratories. *Br. med. J.* **2**, 10.

Report (1962). "A Review of the Medical Services in Great Britain", Report of the Medical Services Review Committee (Chairman Sir Arthur Porritt). London (publisher not given).

Report (1969). "The Use of Antibodies in Animal Husbandry and Veterinary Medicine", Report of DHSS/MAFF Joint Committee (Chairman M.M. Swann), Cmnd 4190. London: HMSO.

Report (1974). "Report of the Committee of Inquiry into the Smallpox in London in March and April 1973" (Chairman P.J. Cox), Cmnd 5626. London: HMSO.

Report (1975). "Report of the Working Party on the Laboratory Use of Dangerous Pathogens" (Chairman Sir George Godber), Cmnd 6054. London: HMSO.

Richmond, S.J., Hilton, A.L., and Clarke, S.K.R. (1972). Chlamydial infection: role of chlamydia subgroup A in non-gonococcal and post-gonococcal urethritis. *Br. J. vener. Dis.* **48**, 437.

Richmond, S.J., Paul, I.D., and Taylor, P.K. (1980). Value and feasibility of screening women attending STD clinics for cervical chlamydial infections. *Br. J. vener. Dis.* **56**, 92.

Robinson, D.A., Edgar, W.M., Gibson, G.L., Matchett, A.A., and Robertson, L. (1979). Campylobacter enteritis associated with consumption of unpasteurized milk. *Br. med. J.* **1**, 1171.

Roebuck, M.O. (1976). Rhinoviruses in Britain 1963–1973. *J. Hyg., Camb.* **76**, 137.

Rountree, P.M. (1949). The phenomenon of lysogenicity in staphylococci *J. gen. Microbiol.* **3**, 153.

Rountree, P.M., and Asheshov, E.H. (1961). Further observations on changes in the phage-typing pattern of phage-type 80/81 staphylococci. *J. gen. Microbiol.* **26**, 111.

Russell, S.M., Benjamin, S.R., Briggs, M., Jenkins, M., Mortimer, P.P., and Payne, S.B. (1978). Evaluation of the single radial haemolysis (SRH) technique for rubella antibody measurement. *J. clin. Path.* **31**, 521.

Selkon, J.B., Stokes, E.R., and Ingham, H.R. (1980). The role of an isolation unit in the control of hospital infection with methicillin-resistant staphylococci. *J. Hosp. Infect.* **1**, 41.

Shipp, C.R., and Rowe, B. (1980). A mechanised microtechnique for salmonella serotyping. *J. clin. Path.* **33**, 595.

Simpson, R.E.H. (1954). Studies on shingles. Is the virus ordinary chickenpox virus? *Lancet ii*, 1299.

Sims, D.G. (1981). A two year prospective study of hospital-acquired respiratory virus infection in paediatric wards. *J. Hyg., Camb.* **86**, 335.

Skirrow, M.B. (1977). Campylobacter enteritis: a "new" disease. *Br. med. J.* **2**, 9.

Smith, J.W.G., and Pollard, R. (1979). Vaccination against influenza: a five-year study in the Post Office. *J. Hyg., Camb.* **83**, 157.

Sompolinsky, D., and Richmond, S.J. (1974). Growth of *Chlamydia trachomatis* in McCoy cells treated with cytochalasin B. *J. appl. Microbiol.* **28**, 912.

Spencely, M., Parker, M.J., Dewar, R.A.D., Miller, D.L., and Moore, B. (1979). The clinical value of microbiological laboratory investigations. *J. Infect.* **1**, 23.

Spicer, C.C. (1954). The generation method of analysis applied to mortality from respiratory tuberculosis. *J. Hyg., Camb.* **52**, 361.

Spicer, C.C. (1959). Influence of some meteorological factors in the incidence of poliomyelitis. *Br. J. prev. soc. Med.* **13**, 139.

Stringer, J., and Maxted, W.R. (1979). Epidemiological evaluation of a phage typing system for group-B streptococci. In "Pathogenic Streptococci: Proceedings of the VIIth International

Symposium on Streptococci and Streptococcal Diseases held in September 1978". Chertsey: Reedbooks.

Taylor, A.G., Harrison, T.G., Dighero, M.W., and Bradstreet, C.M.P. (1979). False positive reactions in the indirect fluorescent antibody test for Legionnaires' disease eliminated by the use of formolised yolk-sac antigen. *Ann. intern. Med.* **90**, 686.

Taylor, J. (1960). The diarrhoeal diseases in England and Wales with special reference to those caused by salmonella, escherichia and shigella. *Bull. Wld Hlth Org.* **23**, 763.

Thomas, M.E.M., and Tillett, H.E. (1975). Sonne dysentery in day schools and nurseries: an eighteen year study in Edmonton. *J. Hyg., Camb.* **71**, 593.

Thomson, Sir A.L. (1975). "Medical Research Council: Half a Century of Medical Research", Vol. 2, "The Programme of the Medical Research Council (UK)". London: HMSO.

Threlfall, E.J., Ward, L.R., Ashley, A.S., and Rowe, B. (1980). Plasmid-encoded trimethoprim resistance in multiresistant epidemic *Salmonella typhimurium* phage types 204 and 193 in Britain. *Br. med. J.* **280**, 1210.

Tobin, J. O'H., Bartlett, C.L.R., Waitkins, S.A., Barrow, G.I., Macrae, A.D. Taylor, A.G., Fallon, R.H., and Lynch, F.R.N. (1981). Legionnaire's disease: further evidence to implicate water storage and distribution systems as sources. *Br. med. J.* **282**, 573.

Tomlinson, A.J.H. (1957). Infected air-borne particles liberated on opening screw-capped bottles. *Br. med. J.* **2**, 15.

Tomlinson, A.J.H., and Mitchell, E.R. (1956). Isolation of poliomyelitis virus in a routine bacteriological laboratory. *Mon. Bull. Min. Hlth Lab. Serv.* **15**, 51.

Topley, W.W.C. (1942). Croonian lecture: the biology of epidemics. *Proc. R. Soc. B* **130**, 337.

Turner, G.C., Ratcliffe, J.G., and Anderson, D. (1976). Penicillinase-producing *Neisseria gonorrhoeae* [Letter to the Editor]. *Lancet ii*, 793.

Wahba, A.H. (1965). Hospital infection with *Pseudomonas aeruginosa*: an investigation by a combined pyocine and serological typing method. *Br. med. J.* **1**, 86.

Wilkinson, A.E. (1954). Studies on the treponemal immobilization test. *Br. J. vener. Dis.* **30**, 38.

Wilkinson, A.E., Seth, A.D., and Rodin, P. (1976). Infection with penicillinase-producing gonococcus. *Br. med. J.* **2**, 1233.

Williams, R.E.O. (1959). Epidemic staphylococci. *Lancet i*, 190.

Williams, R.E.O. (1981). In pursuit of safety. *J. clin. Path.* **34**, 232.

Williams, R.E.O., and Lidwell, O.M. (1957). A protective cabinet for handling infective material in the laboratory. *J. clin. Path.* **10**, 400.

Williams, R.E.O., and Rippon, Joan E. (1952). Bacteriophage typing of *Staphylococcus aureus*. *J. Hyg., Camb.* **50**, 320.

Williams, R.E.O., Rippon, Joan E., and Dowsett, Lynette M. (1953). Bacteriophage typing of strains of *Staphylococcus aureus* from various sources. *Lancet i*, 510.

Wilmers, M.J., Cunliffe, A.C., and Williams, R.E.O. (1954). Type-12 streptococci associated with acute haemorrhagic nephritis. *Lancet i*, 510.

Wilson, G.S. (1948*a*). The public health laboratory service [Milroy Lectures]. *Br. med. J.* **1**, 627 and 677.

Wilson, G.S. (1948*b*). [Presidential address, Section A, Preventive Medicine.] *J. R. sanit. Inst.* **68**, 220.

Wilson, G.S. (1957). Arthur Felix, 3rd April 1887–14th January 1956. *J. Path. Bact.* **73**, 281.

Wilson, G.S., and Atkinson, J.D. (1945). Typing of staphylococci by the bacteriophage method. *Lancet i*, 647.

Yugoslav Typhoid Commission (1962). A controlled field trial of the effectiveness of phenol and alcohol typhoid vaccines. *Bull. Wld Hlth Org.* **26**, 357.

Index

This index incorporates specifically material on pp. i–ix and 1–174; topics referred to in the Appendix (pp. 175–202) are indexed only by general headings.